# Reverse Your Type 2 Diabetes Scientifically

## Get the Facts
## And
## Take Charge of Your Type 2 Diabetes

**Sarfraz Zaidi, MD**

Reverse Your Type 2 Diabetes, Scientifically: Get the Facts And Take Charge of Your Type 2 Diabetes

First Edition, 2014

ISBN-13: 978-1500411695
ISBN-10: 1500411698
Library of Congress Control Number: 2014912365

CreateSpace Independent Publishing Platform
North Charleston, SC

Printed in the United States of America.

## Disclaimer

The information in this book is true and complete to the best of our knowledge. This book is intended only as an informative guide for those wishing to know more about health issues. The information in this book is not intended to replace the advice of a health care provider. The author and publisher disclaim any liability for the decisions you make based on the information contained in this book. The information provided herein should not be used during any medical emergency or for the diagnosis and treatment of any medical condition. In no way is this book intended to replace, countermand or conflict with the advice given to you by your own health care provider. The information contained in this book is general and is offered with no guarantees on the part of the author or publisher. The author and publisher disclaim all liability in connection with the use of this book. The names and identifying details of people associated with events described in this book have been changed. Any similarity to actual persons is coincidental. Any duplication or distribution of information contained herein is strictly prohibited.

# CONTENTS

## *Section 1*

## Get the Facts

# Section 2

## Take Charge of Your Diabetes

# Section 3

## Prevent/Treat/Reverse Complications of Diabetes

## *Section 4*

## **Recipes**

*Section 1*

# Get the Facts

# Introduction

. "Doc, I take my medicines everyday. So why are my blood sugars high?" Peter asked during his first consultation with me. I could sense his utter frustration.

Peter had been under the care of another physician for several years. Initially, he was on one drug, then on two, three and finally on insulin. Despite all of these medicines, he continued to have high blood sugars. He had seen a dietitian and was following her advice most of the time. He also walked everyday, but nothing seemed to be working.

I see diabetics like Peter everyday. What amazes me is how little they know about the root cause of their diabetes. They have been to physicians and dietitians, but haven't heard about insulin resistance-the root cause of Type 2 diabetes, which affects about 95% of diabetics. The other 5% are Type 1 diabetics. It seems no one has explained to them what really causes Type 2 diabetes.

Physicians, dietitians and patients simply follow the drumbeat: diabetes means high blood sugars and control it with diet, exercise and medicines. If one drug does not work, switch to another one, or add another one. They all continue to chase blood sugars like a *wild goose* chase. In the end everyone seems to be frustrated.

Physicians don't have time and often lack in-depth knowledge about insulin resistance. They simply follow the "guidelines" of big medical organizations: which medicines to prescribe, and in which order, which keeps changing every couple of years. Dietitians continue to follow the "guidelines" of their big organization, and follow the algorithms created by these organizations. I call it *robotic* medicine; physicians and dietitians functioning as *robots* of the big medical organizations. Its no surprise that in the end, nothing seem to work and patients bear the consequences of horrendous complications of diabetes.

The purpose of writing this book is to equip you with *scientific* as well as *practical* knowledge about Type diabetes: what works and what does not and why. Then, you can use this information to engage in a meaningful conversation with your physician and take charge of your diabetes.

# Chapter 1

# What Is Type 2 Diabetes?

The majority (about 95%) of diabetic patients are Type 2. In contrast to Type 1 diabetics, most Type 2 diabetics do *not* need insulin shots to manage their diabetes. In Type 2 diabetes, the body is able to produce insulin, but there is resistance to its action. This is known as insulin resistance.

### What is Insulin Resistance?

Insulin is a hormone produced by specialized cells in the pancreas, known as beta-cells. One of the main functions of insulin is to drive glucose from the blood into the cells, especially muscle cells, where it is used as a fuel to produce energy.

Think of the cell as a small room and the blood vessel as a hallway outside of the room. Glucose is a delivery person, running through the hallway trying to enter the room, but the door is closed. Insulin works as the doorman, opening the door for glucose to enter. Insulin must open the door for glucose to enter a cell.

In individuals prone to develop Type 2 diabetes, the doors in the cell wall are difficult to open, as if their hinges are rusty. Consequently, insulin cannot easily open the door. This is called insulin resistance.

### Progression To Type 2 Diabetes

Now, instead of one doorman, you need three or four doormen to pry the door open. In other words, your pancreas produces more and more insulin in response to insulin resistance. This keeps your blood sugar in the normal range for a long time.

If insulin resistance is not treated, as is often the case, the pancreas eventually becomes exhausted and insulin production starts to drop. At this stage, your blood glucose levels start to rise, and you gradually develop prediabetes and then diabetes.

The ability of the pancreas to produce insulin varies from person to person. Some people have a limited ability to produce insulin. They develop diabetes at a younger age—in their twenties and thirties or even in their teens. Others have an extraordinary ability to produce large amounts of insulin. These patients do not develop diabetes until late in life. They may die of a heart attack or stroke before they develop diabetes.

Remember, diabetes is only one of the manifestations of insulin resistance. Other manifestations include prediabetes, high blood pressure, cholesterol disorder, heart disease, stroke, dementia, fatty liver, and a high risk for cancer.

Chapter **2**

# What is Your Type Of Diabetes: Type 1 or Type 2?

In Type 1 diabetes, there is a complete destruction of insulin-producing cells, called beta-cells, in the pancreas. It is an autoimmune process, in which your immune system starts to attack and kill your own insulin-producing cells. Eventually insulin production ceases and diabetes develops.

In Type 2 diabetes, on the other hand, the body is able to produce insulin, but there is *resistance* to the action of insulin. It is a completely different disease from Type 1 diabetes.

### Why Is It Important To Know What Type Of Diabetes You Have?

It is crucial to know what type of diabetes you have, because the appropriate treatment of Type 2 diabetes is completely different from Type 1 diabetes.

While a Type 1 diabetic needs insulin treatment to survive, a Type 2 diabetic does not. A Type 2 diabetic suffers from insulin resistance. Therefore, treatment of a Type 2 diabetic should aim at treating insulin resistance. Insulin does *not* treat insulin resistance.

Unfortunately, many Type 2 diabetics are treated with drugs that stimulate the pancreas to produce more and more insulin and yet nothing is done to treat insulin resistance. The pancreas eventually gets exhausted and cannot keep producing huge amounts of insulin. We can call it pancreatic exhaustion. At that point, these patients are placed on insulin injections to control their blood glucose. Some patients (and surprisingly some physicians) erroneously think that their diabetes is converted from Type 2 to Type 1 and they will have to stay on insulin for the rest of their life.

In fact, if Type 2 diabetics are treated with a strategy to treat their insulin resistance, they do not develop *pancreatic exhaustion* and they do not have to go on insulin. Even those Type 2 diabetics who are already on insulin injections can gradually come off insulin. This is discussed in detail in the chapter on treatment of diabetes.

## Isn't Teenage Diabetes Always Type 1?

In the past, we erroneously used to classify Type 1 diabetes as "Juvenile Onset Diabetes" and Type 2 diabetes as "Adult Onset" or "Maturity Onset." But then we realized that many young people were actually *not* Type 1, but Type 2. As a matter of fact, Type 2 diabetes among teenagers is increasing at an alarming rate, thanks to our culture of fast food and a sedentary lifestyle.

Therefore, now we use the terms Type 1 or Type 2 and don't use the previous, age-related categories. Sadly, I see some physicians still using the old terms.

Presuming someone has Type 1 diabetes based upon their young age can be very misleading.

## Isn't Adult-Onset Diabetes Always Type 2?

Diabetes that develops in adults is almost always Type 2, but rarely it can be Type 1. It happens in people who are thin and worry a lot. Oral medicines do not work in these patients. They need go on insulin to control their blood sugar.

Chapter **3**

# How Can You Tell If Someone Is Type 1 or Type 2?

An endocrinologist, the diabetes expert, can diagnose whether you have Type 1 or Type 2 diabetes based upon clinical information.

Unfortunately, a physician who is not a diabetes specialist may incorrectly categorize the kind of diabetes you have.

**You Are Probably a Type 2 Diabetic If:**

• You are **not** on insulin
• You are on insulin, but in the past you were successfully treated with diabetic pills for several years before you were placed on insulin
• You are on relatively large doses of insulin (usually more than 40 units/day)
• You are obese
• You have high triglycerides (more than 150 mg/dl)
• You have low HDL cholesterol (less than 50mg/dl in females and less than 40 mg/dl in males)
• You have high blood pressure (more than 130/80 mm Hg)
• You have a family history of diabetes, high blood pressure, heart disease, stroke, or high cholesterol

*You Are Probably a Type 1 Diabetic If:*

• You have been on insulin ever since the diagnosis of your diabetes or shortly thereafter (although sometimes your

physician may place you on insulin even though you are a Type 2 diabetic)
• You are on relatively small doses of insulin (usually less than 40 units/day)
• You are thin
• You do not have a family history of diabetes
• You do not have high triglycerides and low HDL cholesterol
• You do not have high blood pressure

## Blood Testing to Categorize the Type of Diabetes:

There is a special blood test that can help categorize whether a person is Type 1 or Type 2. This blood test is known as C-peptide, which is a hormone produced by the pancreas in conjunction with insulin. The blood test for C-peptide should be done one hour after a meal.

Almost all Type 2 diabetic patients have some production of insulin and C-peptide. Actually, many Type 2 diabetics have excessive production of insulin and an elevated level of C-peptide. In contrast, most Type 1 diabetics have no insulin production and, therefore, no C-peptide in their blood.

Rarely, C-peptide is detectable in very small quantities in the early stages of Type 1 diabetes. In these difficult cases, further blood testing, such as anti-islet cell antibodies or anti-GAD antibodies, can be carried out. These antibodies are present in most patients with Type 1 diabetes.

# Chapter **4**

# Insulin May Do More Harm Than Good in Type 2 Diabetes

While insulin is life-saving drug in case of Type 1 diabetes, it may not be the right choice for most Type 2 diabetics. This is why.

In Type 2 diabetic patients, diabetes is one of the manifestations of a seriously harmful disease process in the body called insulin resistance. Simply put, insulin resistance means your own insulin—a hormone naturally produced by the pancreas—becomes less effective in doing its job. In response to this insulin resistance, the pancreas produces more and more insulin. This large amount of insulin is *not* good for your body.

### High Insulin Level Causes High Blood Pressure

A high level of insulin causes high blood pressure. This association between high insulin levels and the development of high blood pressure has been confirmed by several researchers (1).

### High Insulin Level Causes Narrowing of the Blood Vessels

A high level of insulin causes narrowing of the blood vessels, including coronary arteries. In this way, high insulin is associated with coronary artery disease. This association has been documented by several excellent clinical studies—The Helsinki Policeman Study (2), the Paris Prospective Study (3), and the Danish Study (4).

How does insulin cause heart disease? Insulin stimulates smooth muscle cell growth in the walls of arteries and causes thickening and stiffness of arterial walls, which, in turn, contributes to narrowing of blood vessels (5) Hypertension (high blood pressure) itself causes further narrowing of the blood vessels. Narrowed blood vessels lead to heart attacks and strokes.

## High Insulin Level Causes Growth of Tumors, Including Cancer

A high level of insulin also leads to the growth of tumors, benign as well as malignant, because insulin is a growth-promoting hormone. It causes growth of tissues - benign as well as cancerous. Several clinical studies have shown a high prevalence of cancer in people with Insulin Resistance Syndrome. Certain cancers, especially breast cancer, colon cancer and prostate cancer have been linked to insulin resistance. An excellent, large clinical study, known as the Nurses Health Study was published in 2003 in *Diabetes Care* (6). In this study, 111,488 American female nurses who were thirty to fifty-five years old and free of cancer in 1976 were followed through 1996 for the occurrence of Type 2 diabetes and through 1998 for breast cancer. Women with Type 2 diabetes were found to have a higher incidence of breast cancer than those who did not have diabetes.

## Why Insulin May Do More Harm Than Good If You Are A Type 2 Diabetic

Now imagine if a Type 2 diabetic patient, who is already producing a large amount of insulin as a result of insulin resistance, gets  placed on insulin to control elevated blood sugar. It is like adding fuel to the fire, isn't it? That patient is already at high risk for heart disease, hypertension and cancer growth due to high insulin level. Adding more insulin in the form of insulin shots or an insulin pump may control elevated blood sugar, but will increase the risk for high blood pressure, heart attack and cancer. The reverse is also true: If you treat Type 2 diabetes by treating its root cause, the insulin resistance, then you can reduce the risk of heart attack and cancer.

An excellent study from the University of Texas M.D. Anderson Cancer Center in Houston showed that patients with Type 2 diabetes who used insulin were **5 times** more likely to develop pancreatic cancer compared to those who did not use insulin. On the other hand, patients who were on Metformin had a **62% lower risk** for developing pancreatic cancer (7).

Metformin treats insulin resistance. Therefore, it was no surprise that metformin caused a decrease in the risk for pancreatic cancer in this study. In this book, you will learn my comprehensive strategy to treat insulin resistance.

Insulin also causes weight gain, retention of water and low blood sugar (hypoglycemia). Low blood sugar can be life-threatening. Perhaps now you can understand why the *myopic* approach to control blood sugar by insulin can be disastrous in Type 2 diabetic patients.

Caution:

**You must never stop insulin or any other medication, without consulting your health care provider.**

## REFERENCES

1. Manicardi V, Camellini L, Bellodi G, Coscelli C, Ferrannini E. Evidence for an association between high blood pressure and hyperinsulinemia in obese men. *J Clin Endocrinol Metabolism* 1986; 62(6):1302-4.

2. Pyorala K., Savolainen E, Kaukola S, Haapakoski J. Plasma insulin as coronary heart disease risk factor: relationship to other risk factors and predictive value during 9 1/2-year follow-up of the Helsinki Policemen Study. *Acta Med Scand Suppl* 1985; 701:38-52.

3. Eschwege E, Richard JL, Thibult N, et al. Coronary heart disease mortality in relation with diabetes, blood glucose and plasma insulin level. The Paris Prospective Study, ten years later. *Horm Metab Res Suppl* 1985; 15:41–46.

4. Moller LF, Jespersen J. Fasting serum insulin level and coronary heart disease in a Danish cohort: 17-year follow-up. *J Cardiovasc Risk* 1995; 2:235–240.

5. Despres J-P, Lamarche B, et al. Hyperinsulinemia as an independent risk factor for ischemic heart disease. *N Engl J Med* 1996; 334:952–957. Salomaa V, Riley W, Kaark JD, et al. Non–insulin dependent diabetes mellitus and fasting insulin concentrations are associated with arterial stiffness index, the ARIC study. *Circulation* 1995; 91:1432–1443. 239

6. Michels KB, Solomon CG, Hu FB, et al. Type 2 diabetes and subsequent incidence of breast cancer in the Nurses' Health Study. *Diabetes Care* 2003; 26:1752–1758.

7. Li D, Yeung SC, Hassan MM, Konopleva M, Abbruzzese JL. Antidiabetic therapies affect risk of pancreatic cancer. *Gastroenterology.* 2009 Aug;137(2):482-8

Chapter **5**

# Why You Keep Gaining Weight Despite Following The Dietitian's Advice

Many diabetics continue to gain weight despite seeing dietitians and following their advice. Obviously, they get quite frustrated. They bring it up and ask their physician, but don't get a satisfactory answer.

Here are some of the reasons you may gain weight despite following a diet.

### 1. Diet Itself May Be Flawed

Many dietary recommendations are based on out-dated knowledge. Typically, these diets allow too many carbohydrates. That's why many diabetics do not lose weight even when they follow these diets. *More on it in Chapter 11: My New, Scientific Approach To Diabetic Diet.*

### 2. Diabetic Medicines

Many diabetic medicines can cause you to gain weight. *Insulin is the most notorious one.* Other diabetic drugs that often cause weight gain include:

- Glucotrol XL, Glucotrol (glipizide)

- Amaryl (glimepiride)

- Micronase, Diabeta, Glynase (glyburide)

- Diabinese (chlorpropamide)

- Actos ( pioglitazone)

- Avandia (rosiglitazone)

- Prandin (repaglinide)

- Starlix (nateglinide)

## 3. Other Medicines

Diabetics often take several other medicines in addition to their diabetic drugs. Many of these medicines can causes weight gain.

Commonly Used Drugs That Can Cause Weight Gain:

- Steroids such as Deltasone (prednisone), Decadron (dexamethasone)

- Paxil (paroxetine)

- Zyprexa (olanzapine)

- Remeron (mirtazapine)

- Depakote ( valproic acid)

- Thorazine (chlorpromazine)

- Elavil (amitriptyline)

- Depot Medroxyprogesterone Acetate (DMPA)

## 4. Vitamin Deficiencies

Vitamin deficiencies such as Vitamin B12 deficiency and Vitamin D deficiency are common, and can cause weight gain. Low Vitamin D worsens insulin resistance, which can cause weight gain. Low Vitamin B12 leads to low metabolism and consequently weight gain. Vitamin B12 deficiency is particularly common in diabetics on Metformin.

## 5. Under-active Thyroid (Hypothyroidism)

Many diabetics also suffer from under-active thyroid, called hypothyroidism. Often, you may have hypothyroidism, but your physician has not diagnosed it yet. Those patients who have been diagnosed with hypothyroidism are usually prescribed Synthroid, Levoxyl, or Unithroid, which are brand names for Levothyroxine, or T4. Many hypothyroid patients need T3 (Liothyronine), in addition to T4 (Levothyroxine), otherwise they continue to suffer from low metabolism and weight gain.

*To learn more in detail, please refer to my book, "Hypothyroidism and Hashimoto's Thyroiditis."*

## 6. Stress

Stress affects almost every person. Diabetics are no exception. Stress causes weight gain in several ways.

- Stress causes stress eating
- Stress causes hypothyroidism
- Stress causes an increase in cortisol level, which worsens insulin resistance in Type 2 diabetics.
- Stress can cause depression, which can lead to emotional eating and lack of exercise, which culminates in weight gain.

*More on stress and its management in Chapter 10*

# Chapter **6**

# Why Your Blood Sugar Is Higher In The Morning Than The Night Before

Type 2 diabetics often notice their blood glucose is high in the morning although it was better the night before when they went to bed. What happened, you wonder?! I didn't eat anything during the night and my blood glucose went higher. It doesn't make any sense!

There are various reasons why your blood glucose may skyrocket in the morning, which is also called "fasting hyperglycemia."

## 1. Bedtime Snacks

Many diabetics eat a bedtime snack, as they are advised to do so by their dietitian. This is the most common cause of high blood glucose in the morning. A bedtime snack may be appropriate for a type 1 diabetic, but not for most type 2 diabetics, who are overweight to begin with. Stopping or reducing the amount of a bedtime snack may prevent fasting hyperglycemia.

## 2. Increased Production of Glucose by the Liver (Gluconeogenesis)

Normally, the liver produces glucose from fat and protein when you fast. We call it gluconeogenesis. During the night, you don't eat for 8-10 hours, which is a fasting state for the body. Therefore, the liver keeps producing glucose while you are asleep. This is a built-in mechanism to provide a steady supply of glucose to the brain. In fact, a healthy individual, not on any drugs, can fast up to 72-hours and his/her blood glucose will stay normal.

In Type 2 diabetics, this phenomenon of gluconeogenesis gets in *high* gear due to insulin resistance at the level of the liver. Consequently, the liver produces glucose at a much higher rate than it does in non-diabetics, which results in a glucose value in the morning higher than the night before.

You can prevent this exaggerated production of glucose by the liver by treating insulin resistance at the level of the liver. Metformin is one drug that is very effective in treating insulin resistance at the level of the liver. Therefore, if you take Metformin after dinner, and don't eat a bedtime snack, in the morning, your blood glucose will probably not be higher than the night before.

## 3. Dawn Phenomenon

At the crack of dawn, there is a rise in the following hormones in your body: Growth Hormone, Cortisol, Glucagon and Adrenalin, all of which cause an increase in blood glucose. In fact, it is our biologic clock: It's nature telling us to get up and go to work in the fields as our ancestors did for thousands of years. Our modern life style of sleeping through the sunrise is only a couple of hundred years old. It may take thousands of years before our biologic clock adjusts. In the meantime, you can get up early in the morning and go for a walk, or do some exercise at home. This will counteract the morning-rise of blood glucose.

## 4. Not Enough Insulin

Sometimes, a diabetic may *not* be on enough insulin in the early hours of the morning and that gives rise to high morning blood glucose.

Some Type 2 diabetics are on a long-acting insulin such as Lantus (glargine) or Levemir (detemir), which may not be lasting through the early morning hours. Adjusting the dose and/or timing of insulin injection, in consultation with your physician, can take care of this problem.

Some Type 2 diabetics are on an insulin pump these days, which uses only one type of short-acting insulin. Your basal insulin dose may be low in the early morning hours due to the dawn phenomenon. Continuous Glucose Monitoring is very helpful in this regards. Alternatively, you can get up at 3 am and check your blood glucose. Increasing the insulin basal dose, in consultation with your physician, for early morning hours often takes care of this morning hyperglycemia.

## 5. Nighttime Hypoglycemia, Followed By Rebound Hyperglycemia (Somogyi's Effect)

Somogyi's effect is a phenomenon sometimes seen is Type 1 diabetics, but it can also happen in Type 2 diabetics who are on insulin.

Basically, it happens when you are on too much insulin during the nighttime, which causes a low blood glucose, called hypoglycemia. Consequently, your body releases a large amount of Adrenalin and Glucagon, which counter-act hypoglycemia by causing a release of glucose by the liver from the *stored* glucose in the form of glycogen. This process is called Glycogenolysis.

Detecting Somogyi's effect can be quite challenging. Waking up at night with sweats and heart pounding caused by adrenalin release is usually a sign of hypoglycemia. You should obviously check your blood glucose at that time and act accordingly. Sometimes, you may sleep through hypoglycemia. The best way to detect nocturnal hypoglycemia is through Continuous Glucose Monitoring (CGM) or frequent blood glucose monitoring (8-10 times) including getting up at about 3 am to check blood glucose.

## 6. Over-Correcting Night-time Hypoglycemia

Over-Correcting Hypoglycemia at night is more common than Somogyi's effect for causing a high blood glucose in the morning. Hypoglycemia in the middle of the night can be frightening. It is understandable that many diabetics over-react by consuming a large quantity of glucose, which then causes a high glucose in the morning. Please refer to chapter on hypoglycemia on page 225 to learn how to treat hypoglycemia appropriately.

Chapter **7**

# Why Your Blood Sugar Gets Elevated Without Any Apparent Reason

Sometime your blood sugar gets elevated even though you did not change your diet, exercise routine or anti-diabetic medications. You wonder what is going on. Here is a list of various reasons that can increase your blood sugar:

**Stress:**

Both physical and psychological stress can cause an increase in blood glucose. For example, you develop pain in your back, neck, shoulder, or any where else in the body. Then, you may find your blood sugar going up. The stress of an illness such as a bladder infection, flu or even surgery can cause an increase in your blood sugar.

Psychological stress, especially frustration and anger, causes a sharp increase in your blood sugar as well as your blood pressure. Anger is one of the main reasons for an acute heart attack.

The *reverse* is also true. When you are stress-free, your blood sugar comes down nicely. I often hear from my patients that their blood sugars were so much better when they were on a stress-free vacation, even though they were not even very compliant with their diet or did any strenuous exercise.

Stress, physical as well as psychological, causes an increase in adrenaline and cortisol, both of which cause an increase in blood sugar.

## Menses

Some women experience high blood glucose level 3-5 days before or during menses. What causes this increase in blood glucose levels? The answer is progesterone, which is at a high level in your blood before the onset of menses. Progesterone is a hormone produced by the ovaries. It worsens insulin resistance and consequently, raises blood glucose. Progesterone also causes sugar craving from PMS (Premenstrual Syndrome), which further increases blood glucose. In addition, the stress of menses, especially if it is painful, can cause an increase in blood sugar during menses.
So, monitor your blood glucose more frequently before and during menses.

## Medications

Sometimes, your physician adds a medication for some health concern other than diabetes. Certain medications can influence your blood glucose. The common ones are:

### 1. Steroids.

Typically used for arthritis, tendonitis, asthma, or a skin disorder. Many cancer chemotherapy protocols also include steroids. You receive steroids in the form of an injection or pills. Subsequently, you experience a rise in your blood glucose. You wonder what is raising your blood glucose, especially if your physician did not warn you that your diabetes would get out of control with the addition of steroids.

Knowledge of the connection between steroids and a rise in blood glucose can prepare you to deal with your blood glucose escalating after steroid treatments. You should check your blood glucose more frequently after such treatment and make adjustments in the dose of your diabetes medications in consultation with your endocrinologist.

## 2. Beta-Blockers

These drugs are typically used in patients with hypertension and heart disease. Common beta-blockers include: atenolol, propranolol, metoprolol, and sotalol.
These drugs can increase blood sugar and therefore. should be used with caution in patients with diabetes.
Beta-blocker drugs can also complicate hypoglycemia. The body responds to hypoglycemia by producing adrenaline that causes symptoms of hypoglycemia, such as sweating and heart pounding. Beta-blocker drugs interfere with the actions of adrenaline and, therefore, can interfere with the symptoms of hypoglycemia. In other words, you may have hypoglycemia and not be aware of it. So beware and discuss this issue with your physician to make sure that the potential benefits of a beta-blocker drug outweigh its potential risks.

## 3. Birth Control Pills/Hormone Replacement Therapy.

Birth control pills as well as hormone replacement therapy in menopausal women can increase your blood sugar values. So watch your blood sugar closely if you decide to go on birth control pills or hormone replacement therapy.

Chapter **8**

# Why Your Blood Sugar Skyrockets When You Are In The Hospital

I often find my diabetic patients with good control of their diabetes go to the hospital for some acute illness and discover that their diabetes has now soared out of control. Everyone wonders what happened.

A number of factors are usually responsible for this phenomenon.

• Stress (physical and mental) of the acute illness. Imagine being in the busy ER of a hospital while you wait several hours before someone sees you.

• Intravenous fluids. Almost everyone ends up receiving them while in the hospital. Often, they contain glucose.

• Diet. Patients typically receive a diet high in calories as well as high in carbohydrates while in the hospital.

• Interruption of anti-diabetic drugs. Often patients do not receive their anti-diabetic drugs while waiting to be seen, waiting for their tests results, or waiting for admission.

Therefore, next time you are in the hospital, be proactive (without being angry) and pay attention to the common pitfalls mentioned above.

*Section 2*

# Take Charge of Your Diabetes

# Chapter 9

# My Scientific Approach To Treat Type 2 Diabetes

The usual, customary treatment of Type 2 diabetes is *not* very scientific. As I elaborated earlier, the root-cause of Type 2 diabetes is insulin resistance. Doesn't it make sense to treat insulin resistance in order to control Type 2 diabetes?

The customary medicine is well aware of insulin resistance as the root-cause of Type 2 diabetes. But when it comes to treatment, it conveniently *ignores* the root-cause. Instead, it focuses on controlling blood sugars by any drugs, without paying any attention to insulin resistance. Why? Because most anti-diabetic drugs (with the exception of two, which I will discuss in the chapter on Anti-diabetic drugs) do not treat insulin resistance. The anti-diabetic drug industry is huge, and has a lot of muscle. In addition, there is the powerful medical insurance industry.

In my opinion, the pharmaceutical and the medical insurance industries influence, directly or indirectly, the so called *guidelines* of the major medical organizations in the U.S.A. These guidelines tell physicians how to prescribe these anti-diabetic medications for their patients. Why do physicians follow these guidelines? Because physicians in the U.S.A. are fearful of medical lawsuits. There is a common belief among physicians that their best defense against any successful medical litigation is to adhere to the guidelines from big medical organizations.

Perhaps now you understand why customary medicine does *not* focus on treating insulin resistance in the treatment of Type 2 diabetes.

What happens if you do not treat insulin resistance, but try to control blood sugar by whatever anti-diabetic medication has been recommended by big medical organizations? You suffer from the consequences of untreated insulin resistance. These consequences include coronary artery disease, stroke, poor circulation in legs, dementia, cancer growth, kidney disease, peripheral neuropathy and eye disease.

In addition, your insulin resistance gets worse if it stays untreated. Then, you have to keep adding more and more drugs to even control the blood sugars. This is what is called the "step-up" approach. You keep adding more and more steps (drugs) with the passage of time to control your blood sugars. Eventually, most diabetics end up on insulin, and consequently develop many of the complications of insulin resistance and diabetes.

Fifteen years ago, I got the courage to be free of the prison of these medical guidelines. Instead, I focused on treating Type 2 diabetes at its root - insulin resistance. Only then, was I able to not only treat blood sugars effectively, but also to prevent other complications of insulin resistance and diabetes. I call it my scientific approach to treat Type 2 diabetes.

With my approach, once insulin resistance comes under control, you start to reduce the number of medications, even coming off insulin. That's why I like to call this approach the "step-down." You come down (or reduce) the steps (drugs) with the passage of time, instead off adding steps (drugs).

Over the last fifteen years, I have seen some excellent results in my diabetic patients. My new treatment plan, outlined in this book, not only controls diabetes, but also reduces serum triglycerides, increases HDL (good) cholesterol, changes LDL cholesterol from Type B (more dangerous) to Type A (less dangerous), and re-establishes the body's ability to break clots. It accomplishes these major goals by effectively treating insulin resistance—the root cause of these medical disorders. In this way, my new treatment strategy significantly reduces the risk for heart attack, stroke, leg amputation, dementia, kidney disease, eye disease, and other complications of diabetes. Those who already have gone through a coronary angioplasty can stop the vicious cycle of repeated angioplasties. Those who have suffered a stroke can prevent future episodes. Those with memory loss and dementia can prevent further deterioration. Those who have developed an early stage of kidney disease can prevent further progression and avoid ending up on kidney dialysis. Patients with diabetes can now prevent leg amputation and blindness. This certainly has been my clinical experience as the director of the Jamila Diabetes & Endocrine Medical Center.

By using this new treatment strategy, the vast majority of my Type 2 diabetic patients do not need to resort to insulin shots to control their diabetes. Most patients who are already on insulin injections gradually come off insulin. The vast majority of my diabetic patients have *not* required coronary angioplasties, heart bypass surgery, or kidney dialysis. Patients with previous strokes have *not* suffered any further episodes. There have been *no* leg amputations or loss of eyesight in many years.

## My Treatment Strategy To Treat Type 2 Diabetes

My Treatment Strategy To Treat Type 2 Diabetes consists of Five Steps;

- Stress Management
- Proper Nutrition
- Proper Exercise
- Proper Vitamins/Herbs
- Proper Medications, if necessary

I will discuss these five steps in the next five chapters of this book.

First, here a few actual case studies from my practice to illustrate my treatment strategy.

# Mild Type 2 Diabetes

In mild cases of Type 2 diabetes, insulin resistance is the major problem. In response to insulin resistance, the pancreas produces large quantities of insulin. If there is any doubt about insulin production, as may happen if you are not obese, then insulin production can be assessed by checking your C-peptide (or insulin) level with a blood test.

Insulin resistance takes place at three levels: fat, muscle, and liver. Among anti-diabetic drugs, Actos (pioglitazone) treats insulin resistance at the level of fat and muscle and also has mild effects at the level of the liver. The other drug that treats insulin resistance is Metformin, but it primarily treats insulin resistance at the level of the liver only.

Therefore, in mild diabetic patients, I target their insulin resistance by diet, exercise, vitamins, and stress management. In some cases, I may add Actos (pioglitazone).

# Case Study #1

Nadia, a 65 years old female, consulted me for her underactive thyroid (Hypothyroidism). She complained of excessive fatigue. She was on a vegetarian diet. She was on vitamin B12 and Vitamin D supplementation.

Her clinical measurements were as follows:

**Height = 63.5 inches (161 cm)**
**Weight = 104 pounds (47 kg)**
**BMI ( Body Mass Index) = 18 kg/m2** (Normal = 18.5 to 24.9. Overweight when 25 or more, and obesity when 30 or more, according to World Health Organization, WHO)
**Waist Circumference = 23 inches or  58 cm** ( Normal is less than 31.5 inches or 80 cm for women, according to International Diabetes Federation)
**Pulse = 50 beats per minute**

Blood Pressure = 108 / 58 mm Hg

In addition to managing her hypothyroidism, I ordered a 2-hour Oral Glucose Tolerance Test.

## Results of 2-hour Oral Glucose Tolerance Test

|  | Baseline | 1 hour | 2 hour |
|---|---|---|---|
| Blood Glucose (Normal Range) | 77 mg/dl ( < than 100) | 199 mg/dl (75 - 200) | 237 mg/dl (75 - 140) |

This test showed that she had diabetes, as evidenced by the 2-hour blood glucose level above 200 mg/dl, although her fasting blood glucose was in the normal range.

I placed her on my Diabetes Treatment Plan, which included Stress Management, proper diet, exercise and vitamins. I decided *not* to place her on any anti-diabetic medication, as she was a mild case of Type 2 diabetes.

Just with life-style changes and vitamins, she achieved an excellent control of her Type 2 diabetes and insulin resistance, as evidenced by HbA1c, HDL2, LDL-Pattern, and lowering of her insulin level, all of which are in the normal range. She feels great and wants to share her experience with other diabetics, in order to help them.

## Diabetes Progress Report

|  | Baseline | 9 months | 15 Months | Normal Range |
|---|---|---|---|---|
| Fasting Blood Glucose (mg/dl) | 77 | 87 | 81 | Less than 100 |

| HbA1c | Not Done | 5.7% | 5.4% | 5.6 % or less |
|---|---|---|---|---|
| HDL Cholesterol (mg/dl) | 53 | 65 | 72 | More than 40 |
| HDL 2 Cholesterol (mg/dl) | Not Done | 14 | 18 | More than 15 |
| Triglycerides (mg/dl) | 118 | 52 | 41 | Less than 150 |
| LDL Cholesterol (mg/dl) | 120 | 94 | 88 | Less than 100 |
| LDL Pattern | Not Done | B | A | A |

Fasting Blood Glucose in mg/dl
HDL = HDL Cholesterol in mg/dl
HDL2 = HDL2 Cholesterol in mg/dl
Trig = Triglycerides in mg/dl
LDL = LDL Cholesterol in mg/dl
Pattern = LDL Pattern
HbA1c = Hemoglobin A1c

## Lessons to Learn

- Even thin people can develop Type 2 diabetes.

- You can be diabetic even if your fasting blood glucose is in the normal range.

- The best test to diagnose diabetes is a 2-hour Oral Glucose Tolerance Test (OGTT). This test diagnoses diabetes several years before any other blood test.

- I would have missed the diagnosis of diabetes in this patient, if I did not order a 2-hour Oral Glucose Tolerance Test (OGTT).

# Case Study #2

Zara, a fifty-four-year-old woman with a history of elevated triglycerides and elevated blood glucose levels, came to see me for her fatigue. Her mother and two brothers all had Type 2 diabetes.

I gave her a two-hour oral glucose tolerance test (OGTT) with the following results:

### Results of 2-hour Oral Glucose Tolerance Test

|  | Baseline | 1 hour | 2 hour |
|---|---|---|---|
| Blood Glucose<br><br>(Normal Range) | 111 mg/dl<br><br>(< than 100) | 279 mg/dl<br><br>(75 - 200) | 247 mg/dl<br><br>(75 - 140) |

This test confirmed that she indeed was diabetic. She was not obese. Therefore, I checked her C-peptide level, which was high, indicating she was producing large amounts of insulin in response to insulin resistance.

I placed her on my 5 step plan to treat her insulin resistance and diabetes. Zara's diabetes is under excellent control as evidenced by her hemoglobin A1c level which has stayed in the non-diabetic range over the past thirteen years.

Three years ago, Zara developed an infection in her knee after an orthopedic surgeon gave her a steroid injection into her knee for degenerative arthritis. Zara was on intravenous antibiotics for six weeks. Although her infection got cured, her knee joint got destroyed from the infection. Consequently, she cannot walk much. Despite severe limitation on her walking, Zara continues to have an excellent control of her diabetes and insulin resistance.

## Diabetes Progress Report

|  | Initial | 4 years | 11 years | 13 years |
|---|---|---|---|---|
| Fasting blood Glucose (mg/dl) | 111 | 85 | 83 | 92 |
| HbA1c | Not Done | 5.5% | 5.8% | 5.7% |
| HDL Cholesterol (mg/dl) | 55 | 65 | 57 | 59 |
| HDL 2 Cholesterol (mg/dl) | Not Done | 26 |  | 14 |
| Triglycerides (mg/dl) | 101 | 61 | 63 | 76 |
| LDL Cholesterol (mg/dl) | 109 | 69 | 177 | 144 |
| LDL Pattern | Not Done | A |  | A |

*Fasting Blood Glucose in mg/dl*

*HDL = HDL Cholesterol in mg/dl*
*HDL2 = HDL2 Cholesterol in mg/dl*
*Trig = Triglycerides in mg/dl*
*LDL = LDL Cholesterol in mg/dl*
*Pattern = LDL Pattern*
*HbA1c = Hemoglobin A1c*

Zara has not developed any complications of diabetes/insulin resistance over the last thirteen years. At the age of sixty seven, she continues to enjoy good physical health except difficulty in walking due to her bad knee. She has learned how to deal with the stress of daily living. That's why her diabetes/ insulin resistance stays under excellent control even without any exercise.

Zara wants to share her great experience with others who suffer from Type 2 diabetes.

## Lessons to Learn

- The Oral Glucose Tolerance Test is superior to a fasting blood glucose test in diagnosing early Type 2 diabetes.

- Your body produces a large amount of insulin in the early stages of Type 2 diabetes.

- With my 5-step approach, you can achieve excellent long-term control of your Type 2 diabetes/insulin resistance. Then you don't have keep adding more and more drugs.

- If for some reason, you are unable to exercise, as happened with this patient, you still can achieve excellent control of Type 2 diabetes/insulin resistance, if you faithfully stick to the other four steps of my approach.

# Moderate Type 2 Diabetes

When Type 2 diabetes is not diagnosed for a period of time, it progresses to a more advanced stage. It is evidenced by a higher hemoglobin A1c level than individuals in mild cases. These patients often have developed some complications of diabetes by the time their diabetes is diagnosed.

As in mild cases, insulin resistance is the major problem in moderate cases of Type 2 diabetes. There is still enough insulin production by the pancreas. Therefore, I focus on treating insulin resistance in these individuals. To this end, I use my 5-step approach— stress management, diet, exercise, vitamins, and medications.

# Case Study #3

Liz, a sixty-eight-year-old female, consulted me for the management of her newly diagnosed type 2 diabetes.

She had a history of Pre-diabetes, and was on Metformin per her primary care physician. Then, she was found to have an elevated fasting blood glucose of 149 mg/dl and HBA1C of 7.0 %, both of which indicated that she had become diabetic.

At that point, she consulted me. She complained of excessive fatigue. Her clinical measurements were as follows:

**Weight = 208 pounds (94 kg)**
**Height = 63.75 inches (162 cm)**
**BMI ( Body Mass Index) = 36 kg/m2** (Normal = 18.5 to 24.9. Overweight when 25 or more, and obesity when 30 or more, according to World Health Organization, WHO)
**Waist Circumference = 41 inches or 104 cm** ( Normal is less than 31.5 inches or 80 cm for women, according to International Diabetes Federation)
**Blood Pressure = 140 / 70 mm Hg**
**Pulse = 80 beats per minute**

According to these measurements, she had obesity and mild hypertension.

I ordered a 2-hour Oral Glucose Tolerance Test (OGTT) to confirm her diagnosis of diabetes, as well as to assess the status of her insulin production.

## Results of 2-hour Oral Glucose Tolerance Test

|  | Baseline | 1 hour | 2 hour |
|---|---|---|---|
| Blood Glucose (Normal Range) | 126 mg/dl (< than 100) | 291 mg/dl (75 - 200) | 214 mg/dl (75 - 140) |
| Blood insulin (Normal Range) | 17 mU/L (3 - 28) | 83 mU/L (29 - 112) | 114 mU/L (22 - 79) |

Results of the OGTT clearly showed that her prediabetes had progressed to Type 2 diabetes. She also had high levels of insulin, which typically is the case in the early stages of Type 2 diabetes. High insulin levels happen as a result of insulin resistance. Obviously Metformin alone was *ineffective* in treating her insulin resistance, and preventing her from becoming diabetic.

In addition to elevated blood glucose levels, she also had low HDL and high triglycerides for a long time. Her primary care physician had placed her on Simvastatin (generic for Zocor) to treat her cholesterol disorder. Simvastatin is a Statin drug, and there are several others such as Atorvastatin (Lipitor), Rosuvastatin (Crestor), Pravastatin (Pravachol) and Lovastatin (Mevacor).

When she came to see me, her Lipid panel was as follows:

| | Patient's Result | Normal Range |
|---|---|---|
| HDL Cholesterol | 50 mg/dL | More than 40 |
| HDL 2 Cholesterol | 12 mg/dL | More than 15 |
| Triglycerides | 164 mg/dL | Less than 150 |
| LDL Cholesterol | 98 mg/dL | Less than 100 |
| LDL Pattern | A/B | A |

Her total HDL level was in the normal range, but her HDL2, which is the most-protective cholesterol, was indeed low. Therefore, you should have your HDL2 level checked, if you truly want to know your most-protective cholesterol level. Low HDL2 meant she was having insulin resistance, despite being on Metformin and Simvastatin.

Her triglycerides level was high and LDL pattern was A/B, both of which indicated that her insulin resistance was not treated, despite being on Metformin and Simvastatin. Her LDL quantity was less than 100 mg/dL, which was due to Simvastatin. This case study clearly illustrates that Simvastatin (and other statins) simply lowers LDL cholesterol, but does not treat insulin resistance. Even Metformin alone does not treat insulin resistance effectively.

She was obese with a waist-line of 41 inches. Her Blood pressure was mildly elevated as 140/70. She was also experiencing a lot of fatigue.

Management:

I diagnosed her with Insulin Resistance Syndrome, and placed her on my 5-step treatment program for Type 2 diabetes and insulin resistance.

I also diagnosed her underactive thyroid (hypothyroidism), which was missed by her primary care physician, because her TSH was in the so-called normal range: A common pitfall. For more details, please refer to my book, "Hypothyroidism And Hashimoto's Thyroiditis."

Over a 9-month period, she lost 45 lbs. Now, she has a lot of energy and feels great. She wants to share her great experience with others who suffer from Type 2 diabetes.

### Diabetes Progress Report

|  | Baseline | 3 months | 6 months | 9 months |
|---|---|---|---|---|
| Fasting Blood Glucose (mg/dl) | 149 | 98 | 88 | 93 |
| HbA1c | 7.0% | 5.7% | 5.6% | 5.6% |
| HDL Cholesterol (mg/dl) | 50 | 57 | 67 | 74 |
| HDL 2 Cholesterol (mg/dl) | 12 | 16 | 20 | 21 |
| Triglycerides (mg/dl) | 164 | 100 | 93 | 88 |
| LDL Cholesterol (mg/dl) | 98 | 81 | 83 | 97 |
| LDL Pattern | A/B | A | A | A |

Fasting Blood Glucose in mg/dl
HDL = HDL Cholesterol in mg/dl
HDL2 = HDL2 Cholesterol in mg/dl
Trig = Triglycerides in mg/dl
LDL = LDL Cholesterol in mg/dl
Pattern = LDL Pattern
HbA1c = Hemoglobin A1c

As you can see, her diabetes got in the reverse gear, as evidenced by her fasting blood glucose as well as HbA1c coming in the <u>non-diabetic</u> range within three months of treatment. These levels continue to be in the <u>non-diabetic</u> range at 9 months, at the time of writing this book.

In addition, HDL2 cholesterol and triglycerides improved tremendously. Her LDL pattern changed to A from A/B. All of these changes clearly indicate that her Insulin Resistance came under excellent control within 3 months, and continues to be under excellent control at 6 months. She feels great and wants to share her experience with other diabetics in order to help them.

**Lessons to Learn:**

1. Metformin alone usually does not prevent progression from prediabetes to diabetes, as is obvious in this case. This has been our experience at the Jamila Diabetes and Endocrine Medical Center. In a landmark clinical study (1), DPP (Diabetes Prevention Program) in the US, researchers found that diet and exercise was much more effective than Metformin in preventing progression from prediabetes to diabetes (58% versus 31%).

2. The best measurement for HDL cholesterol is HDL2 and *not* total HDL.

3. Statin drugs lower your LDL cholesterol, but have no significant effect on HDL or triglycerides or insulin resistance.

4. It is important to check LDL pattern, in addition to its quantity. Pattern B is associated with insulin resistance, and carries a

much higher risk for cardiovascular events than Pattern A. Pattern A/B carries an intermediate risk.

5. An increase in HDL2, a decrease in triglycerides and a shift from LDL pattern B to A, *signifies* that insulin resistance is coming under control.

6. A comprehensive approach aimed at stress management, diet, exercise, vitamins and proper oral medications can put your Type 2 diabetes into reverse gear, even into the non-diabetic range.

7. Physicians often miss the diagnosis of Underactive thyroid (hypothyroidism), as they stay focused on TSH (thyroid Stimulating Hormone) for the diagnosis of hypothyroidism. In a chronic disease, such as diabetes, the active thyroid hormone (T3) goes down in the entire body except the pituitary gland, where TSH is produced. In  this way, your pituitary gland is healthy, but the rest of the body is hypothyroid. For more details, refer to my book, "Hypothyroidism And Hashimoto's Thyroiditis."

## Severe Type 2 Diabetes

When Type 2 diabetes is not diagnosed for an even longer period of time, it progresses to a more advanced stage as evidenced by markedly elevated hemoglobin A1c of more than 8%.

In severe cases of diabetes, in addition to insulin resistance, there is a relative *decrease* in insulin production by the pancreas.

This decrease in insulin production is due to two reasons:

1. Glucose-toxicity: High blood glucose levels have a toxic effect on the insulin-producing cells in the pancreas itself. This phenomenon is called glucose-toxicity. It is *reversible* with good control of blood glucose levels.

2. Lipo-toxicity: Patients with insulin resistance have a high level of free fatty acids, which are toxic to the insulin-producing cells in the pancreas. This phenomenon is known as lipotoxicity. Free fatty acids are usually measured in research laboratories and *not* in a typical clinical setting. In clinical practice, we use the serum triglyceride level as an assessment of the amount of free fatty acids. If your triglyceride level is more than 150 mg/dl, you have a high level of free fatty acids.

**In summary**, there are three fundamental defects in severe cases of Type 2 diabetic patients:

- Insulin resistance in the muscle and fat
- Insulin resistance in the liver
- Decrease in the production of insulin by the pancreas *relative* to the insulin resistance. As a general rule, the longer the duration of diabetes, the lesser is the insulin production.

All three of these defects must be addressed to treat diabetes effectively. Picture a triangular enclosure for the angry beast we call diabetes. You can't keep it under control if you secure only one or two sides of the triangle. It will continue to go on a rampage wherever it finds an opening. You have to control all three sides of this triangle to keep it contained. I call it the treatment triangle for diabetes.

# Case Study #4

Alfredo, a forty-two-year-old male, is a good example of a patient with severe diabetes who achieved excellent control using my treatment approach.

Alfredo consulted me for his newly diagnosed diabetes. Over the past year, he had experienced excessive thirst, frequent urination, and blurry vision, but he did not seek medical advice. Finally, he went to a local hospital where they found his non-fasting blood glucose to be markedly elevated at 465 mg/dl. He was sent home on Glucophage (Metformin.) A couple of weeks later, he came to see me.

Alfredo's father, mother, and two grandparents all had Type 2 diabetes. His maternal grandfather had high blood pressure, coronary heart disease, and a stroke.

Alfredo's clinical measurements were as follows:

**Weight = 152 pounds (69 Kg)**
**Height = 67.0 inches (170 cm)**
**BMI ( Body Mass Index) = 24 kg/m2** (Normal = 18.5 to 24.9. Overweight when 25 or more, and obesity when 30 or more, according to World Health Organization, WHO)
**Blood Pressure = 105 / 70 mm Hg**
**Pulse = 80 beats per minute**

## *Laboratory Results*

**Fasting blood glucose = 228 mg/dl** (should be 70–100 mg/dl)
**HbA1c = 12.2%** (should be less than 5.7%)
**Triglycerides = 155 mg/dl** (should be less than 150 mg/dl)
**HDL Cholesterol = 37 mg/dl** (should be more than 40 mg/dl in males)
**LDL Cholesterol = 183 mg/dl Type B** (should be less than 100 mg/dl and Type A pattern)
**ALT = 66 u/l** (should be less than 30 u/l) (ALT, short for alanine aminotransferase, is a blood test for liver function. An elevated ALT means that your liver function is abnormal.)

## *Diagnosis*

In view of his elevated triglycerides, low HDL cholesterol, Type B LDL cholesterol, and his family history, I suspected that Alfredo's diabetes was Type 2 and that he was suffering from Insulin Resistance Syndrome. However, in view of his symptoms of excessive thirst and urination and the fact that he was not overweight, I wanted to make sure that he did not have Type 1 diabetes. So I ordered a C-peptide level, which turned out to be 2.0 ng/ml (normal range = 0.8–3.1 ng/ml) indicating that indeed he had Type 2 diabetes.

His elevated ALT indicated liver inflammation from fatty liver, a complication of insulin resistance and Type 2 diabetes. More on it in chapter 28: Fatty Liver in Diabetics on page 275.

## Management

I educated Alfredo about diabetes and Insulin Resistance Syndrome and placed him on my 5-step treatment approach.

Over the past <u>ten</u> years, he continues to have excellent control of his diabetes. His A1C has stayed under 6.5%, often under 6.0% indicating he has his Type 2 diabetes has regressed and is staying in the non-diabetic range.

Good control of insulin resistance also shifted his LDL pattern from pattern B (really harmful) to pattern A (less harmful), and has remained pattern A over the last <u>ten</u> years.

With control of insulin resistance, his HDL went up from 37 mg/dl to 53 within a matter of months, and has stayed higher than 50 over the last ten years. His last HDL reading was 68 mg/dl.

His ALT came down to a normal level within one month and has stayed normal for the last <u>ten</u> years.

Alfredo enjoys great physical and mental health. He has not developed any complications of diabetes/insulin resistance over the last ten years. He is still very active in his demanding career as well as personal life, but he has learned how to manage the stress of daily living, which is the key to his long-term success with his diabetes/insulin resistance management.

He feels great and wants to share his experience with other diabetics.

# Diabetes Progress Report

| | Baseline | 1 month | 5 months | 10 months | 2 years | 4 years | 10 years |
|---|---|---|---|---|---|---|---|
| FBG (mg/dl) | 228 | 90 | 113 | 105 | 99 | 116 | 127 |
| HbA1c | 12.2% | 9.0% | 5.7% | 5.6% | 5.3% | 5.9% | 6.4% |
| HDL (mg/dl) | 37 | | | 53 | | 55 | 68 |
| HDL 2 | | | | 14 | | | 17 |
| Trig (mg/dl) | 155 | | | 87 | | 103 | 77 |
| LDL (mg/dl) | 183 | | | 50 | | 69 | 54 |
| Pattern | B | A | A | A | | | A |
| 25 OH Vitamin D (ng/ml) | | | 42 | | | 57 | |

FBG= Fasting Blood Glucose in mg/dl
HDL = HDL Cholesterol in mg/dl
HDL2 = HDL2 Cholesterol in mg/dl
Trig = Triglycerides in mg/dl
LDL = LDL Cholesterol in mg/dl
Pattern = LDL Pattern
HbA1c = Hemoglobin A1c

## Lessons to Learn

- My 5-step approach can reverse/regress even severely uncontrolled Type 2 diabetes into the non-diabetic range.

- Effective control of insulin resistance is the best way to increase your HDL (good) cholesterol, and to change LDL pattern from B (more harmful) to A (less harmful).

- Severely uncontrolled Type 2 diabetes can cause liver damage, which is reversible with an excellent control of insulin resistance.

- You can prevent all complications of diabetes and insulin resistance, with an excellent control of insulin resistance.

- Excellent control of insulin resistance prevents you from going on insulin therapy.

## How to Come Off Insulin Treatment in Type 2 Diabetes

As I elaborated earlier, many Type 2 diabetic patients end up on insulin because their insulin resistance is not effectively treated. Insulin may control blood sugars, but these patients develop complications of insulin resistance, which includes coronary artery disease, stroke, poor circulation in legs, dementia, cancer growth, kidney disease, peripheral neuropathy and eye disease.

## Case Study #5

Susan, a 67 years old Caucasian female, consulted me for her diabetes management.

She was diagnosed with type 2 diabetes about thirty one years ago. In addition, she had high blood pressure, low HDL cholesterol, high triglycerides, abdominal obesity and underactive thyroid. For the past several years, she was under the care of an endocrinologist.

Four years ago, her endocrinologist stopped her Metformin, which she was on for several years, and switched her to Byetta. She developed severe nausea and vomiting. Her endocrinologist switched her from Byetta to Bydureon, but nausea and vomiting continued. She also developed lethargy and depression.

About one year ago, she was hospitalized with blood glucose in the 500 range. At that point, her endocrinologist placed her on two insulins: Levemir and Novolog. A few months later, Victoza was added. Now, she was taking *five* daily injections of diabetic medicines, but her diabetes was still out of control. She was checking her BG (Blood Glucose) 4 times a day. Her pre-meal blood glucose readings were around 150-200 and post-meal blood glucose readings were around 150. In addition, she would have a hypoglycemic episode every 1-2 weeks.

She had developed diabetic retinopathy, requiring multiple Laser treatments. She had also developed Diabetic nephropathy and was seeing a nephrologist. Her urinary Microalbumin/Creatinine was **388** one year ago, rose to **796** nine months ago. It had climbed to **978**, when she came to see me.

She was on a long list of medications and supplements as follows:

Levemir Flexpen (insulin detemir)
Novolog Flexpen (insulin aspart)
Victoza (liraglutide) = 0.6 mg twice a day
Losartan = 100 mg a day
Hydrochlorothiazide = 12.5 mg a day
Pravastatin = 80 mg a day
Synthroid (levothyroxine) = 150 mcg a day
Vitamin B12-folic acid = 1,000-400 mcg
Vitamin C (ascorbic acid) = 250 mg
Vitamin D3 = 2,000 unit

Biotin
Magnesium = 250 mg tablet
Co Q10-red yeast rice = 60-600 mg
Fish Oil = 360-1,200 mg

I spent a long time with her, educating her about my 5-step approach to Type 2 diabetes and insulin resistance syndrome. I stopped her insulins, Levemir as well as Novolog. I also stopped Victoza.

At four months, she had excellent control of her diabetes. She felt much better. She had lost 5 Lbs.

## Diabetes Progress Report

|  | Baseline | 4 months |
|---|---|---|
| FBG (mg/dL) | 157 | 109 |
| HbA1c | 8.2% | 6.6% |
| HDL (mg/dL) | 40 | 46 |
| Triglycerides (mg/dL) | 262 | 207 |
| LDL (mg/dL) | 72 | 68 |
| Microalbumin/Cr (mcg/mg) | 978 | 430 |

FBG= Fasting Blood Glucose in mg/dl
HDL = HDL Cholesterol in mg/dl
LDL = LDL Cholesterol in mg/dl
HbA1c = Hemoglobin A1c

Susan is thrilled to have such good control of her diabetes, and to be off insulin as well as Victoza injections. She is especially excited to see that her kidney disease is getting better.

She feels great and wants to share her experience with other diabetics in order to help them.

## Lessons To Learn

- If you don't treat insulin resistance, you will develop complications of diabetes. This patient developed eye disease and kidney disease despite taking multiple medications.

- If you don't treat insulin resistance, you will eventually end up on insulin therapy, which may or may not control your blood sugars. As you can clearly see, this patient was on two types of insulin as well as Victoza, but her diabetes was still out of control, and her kidney disease was getting worse.

- By effectively treating her insulin resistance, she achieved a much better control of blood sugars within a matter of a few months.

*Please also refer to case Study #6 to learn how to come off insulin therapy, in Chapter 22: Kidney Disease in Diabetics on page 247*

These cases studies clearly illustrate that insulin resistance, the root cause of Type 2 diabetes, must be treated in Type 2 diabetic patients. Only then you can stop the progression and often reverse/regress the course of Type 2 diabetes.

*In the next Five Chapters, I elaborate on my 5-step treatment strategy to treat Type 2 diabetes by targeting insulin resistance.*

## References

1. Knowler WC, Barrett-Connor E, Fowler SE, Hamman RF, Lachin JM, Walker EA, Nathan DM. Reduction in the incidence of type 2 diabetes with lifestyle intervention or metformin. *N Engl J Med.* 2002;346:393–403.

Chapter **10**

# My Unique Approach To Stress Management

Many diabetics know their blood sugar gets elevated when they are under stress, even though their eating habits didn't change at all. They also know their elevated blood sugar comes down with the release of stress.

Even subtle stress can elevate your blood glucose levels. For example, some diabetics get so preoccupied by their blood sugar readings that they stress themselves out. As a result, their blood sugar reading starts to escalate. Then, they get more stressed out and a vicious cycle sets in.

### Emergency Management Of Stress

When faced with an acute, stressful situation, do the following:

**Pause.** Take time-out. Don't *say* or *do* anything.

Feel the *emotion* rising inside you. Don't *suppress* it. At the same time, don't get *consumed* by the emotion. Instead, start *counting*. See how long does it takes for the *emotion* to subside.

Be acutely aware of your surroundings: the *objects* and the *space* in which objects are; the *sounds* and the *silence*, which remains in the background of all sounds; the *movements* and the *stillness,* which remains in the background of all movements. Remember 3-S': Space, Silence and Stillness.

Be aware of your *breathing*.

Once emotion has settled down, use *logic* and *analyze* the entire situation as a *third party*, from a *neutral ground*. You will be amazed to see that your emotion was way *out of proportion* to the actual situation. Then, completely *let go* of whatever happened. Be aware of the nagging *inner voice* that wants you to keep *festering* over "what happened." Simply *laugh* at it and *move* on.

Go out for a walk in your neighborhood park, or even in your backyard.

Look at nature: the trees, the sky, the flowers, the stars, the sunset, the sunrise. Also, be aware of the *space* in which every thing is.

Listen to nature: the birds, the crickets, the dogs. Also, be aware of the *silence* which is always there. Sounds come and go, but silence is always there.

Use your sense of *smell* to be aware of various fragrances.

**Decompress On A Regular Basis**

Do certain activities to *decompress* your stress on a regular basis so it does not build up to a *crisis* point. Here are some suggestions:

Do some *stretches* everyday or better yet, several times a day, just a few minutes of stretches at a time, that's all.

Every now and then pay attention to your breathing, just for a minute or so. Also, do deep breathing for a minute or so, a couple of times during the day.

Go for a walk on a daily basis.

# Stress Management At Its Roots

You may already know some of the *advice* I just gave. It does work, but only *temporarily*. Often, you continue to struggle with the *stress of daily life*.

In this section, we take a *deeper* look at *stress*. We investigate what stress really is, what is its root cause and how you can be free of stress, once and for all

## What Is Stress?

You are finally home after a long day at work. It's time to relax. You ease yourself into your new sofa. Without even realizing it, soon your mind is back at work. You think about how your day went: that annoying customer; the ungrateful, greedy boss; the jealous, selfish co-worker.

Finally, your husband arrives exhausted and complaining about all of the annoyances he went through during the day. He also expresses his worries about the bleak economic future for the family.

On the answering machine, you hear a reminder about your appointment the next day with your doctor to discuss the result of your biopsy. What if the biopsy turns out to be cancerous? A wave of shivers runs through your body. In bed, you toss and turn, but sleep is miles away. At 2 am, you pop some sleeping pills and manage to get four hours of sleep.

At the physician's office your biopsy report is fine, but your weight is up, blood pressure is high and your blood sugar is also borderline high. Later, on the way back to work, you can't help but think about your dad, who couldn't walk in his old age due to a stroke caused by his high blood pressure and your mom, who lost her eyesight because of diabetes.

Suddenly, you feel your heart pounding, chest tightening, and body losing all of its strength. Next, you wake up in the emergency room at a hospital ...........

The *stress of daily living* has horrendous consequences. Everyone suffers from it to a certain degree. People reluctantly accept it. "This is part of life and there's nothing you can do about it." In this way, they *rationalize* their stressful living.

Is it possible to be free of stress? Don't you need to fully understand stress before you can be free of it? Stress comes in many forms. For the sake of discussion, I divide stress into two types:

- Outer stress
- Inner Stress

## Outer Stress

Outer stress is what we generally refer to when we talk of stress. This is the stress due to an external factor, often out of our control, such as loss of a loved one, losing a job, missing a flight.

These are basically situations which keep happening, one after another. There are brief periods when we get some relief. You may think, "Ah! Finally I have no stress," but before you know it, some other stressful situation arrives.

For example, after years of hard work, you finally have the ideal job you always wanted. You have a nice house, a nice car and a wonderful family. Then one day, you have a serious car accident and spend the next several weeks on crutches. Finally, you're back at work, but find out that your company is in financial trouble. Soon, you're laid off. Lack of a job, obviously, creates a huge stress. A few months later, your wife is diagnosed with cancer. While she's undergoing chemotherapy, you find out you need heart bypass surgery. In the meantime, your teenager is having problems with teachers. You find yourself a frequent visitor to the principal's office.

Another example: You finally reach the retirement that you've been dreaming of for years. Soon after retirement, you discover that you have prostate cancer, for which you undergo surgery. As a complication of surgery, you can no longer control your urine. A few months later, your wife falls, breaks her hip and ends up in the hospital. In the meantime, your daughter calls to let you know that she is going through a divorce and will need financial aid from you.

Well, you get the idea of the many types of outer stresses that we encounter in our lives!

## Inner Stress

Inner stress, on the other hand, is a different animal. It's there all the time. With few exceptions, everyone is suffering from it. It stays with you wherever you go.

What is this inner stress? It's the feeling of restlessness, agitation, emptiness, worthlessness, sadness, boredom, frustrations, annoyances, anger, hate, jealousy, insecurity, guilt, fear, nervousness and anxiety.

Where does this inner stress come from? If you pay close attention, you'll find that this inner stress comes from your own *inner voice*, the voice in your head that never stops even though you have nothing to solve. Often, you're completely unaware of it. It's like your mind is on *autopilot.* In other words, you think constantly. You have a busy mind that never stops. Thoughts, then trigger emotions and create emotional stress for you. Therefore, it is logical to conclude that *emotional thoughts* are the root cause of your inner stress.

## What Is The Basis Of Thoughts?

Where do thoughts come from? While pondering over this question one day, I made a simple, yet profound observation. <u>We humans, always think in terms of a language</u>. For example, if you know English and no other language, you will always think in English, not in Chinese, French or Hindi. Just observe it right now, yourself.

In order to think, you need to know a language. Therefore, language is the basis of thoughts.

## What Is The Basis Of Language?

Obviously, the next question is where does the language come from? You are not born with it, right? You learn it as you grow up in a society. You learn it from your parents, teachers, siblings, friends and various tools such as books, electronic devices and sometimes, certain other techniques.

## What Is A Language?

Let's use common sense and explore what is a language? It is a *means* to communicate with each other. A language is comprised of words, right? And each word has a <u>concept</u> attached to it. In reality, every word is a <u>sound</u>. For example, listen to a language you don't know. All you will hear is sounds: sounds that make no sense. In order to make sense, you need to know the concepts attached to the sounds. In this way, we can say that a word consists of a <u>sound </u>and an attached <u>concept</u>. Even written language has <u>concepts</u> attached to words. Even Sign language has <u>concepts</u> attached to signs.

## What Is The Basis Of Concepts?

Let's use common sense and find out where concepts come from. Concepts are the creation of a society, aren't they? When you grow up in a society, your parents teach you the language of that society. They utter a sound and point to a person or some object. They keep repeating it until you make a *connection* between that sound and the person or object. For example: As a baby, you hear the sound Mama as your mother points a finger towards herself. After a lot of repetition, you make a connection between the sound and the person. She is no longer another life form, but Mama. She provides you with food, comfort and warmth. You get *attached* to her. Later, she provides you with toys, gifts, friends, cupcakes, cookies, money and so on. You get more and more attached to "your Mama."

As you grow up in a society, you are *bombarded* with concepts that society has created, such as the concepts of success, failure, achievement, money, fame, desirable, undesirable, morality, etiquette, responsibility, culture, customs, religion, nationality, past, future, security, etc. Based on these concepts, certain thoughts may arise, such as thoughts of losing, being a failure, an outcast, punishment, suffering, how one should and shouldn't behave, why did it happen, why it didn't happen, what if, why me, why not me, etc. All of these thoughts trigger emotions such as fear, anger, sadness, jealousy, guilt. This is how your thoughts create a huge amount of stress for you.

## Who Is Thinking?

If you pay attention, you realize it is always "I" who judges others, who blames others, who is afraid of this and that etc. It is the "I" who is thinking. Therefore, it is the "I" who is at the <u>root</u> of all of your stress. Who is this "I"? We need to figure this out, if we truly want to be free of stress.

## The Virtual "I"

Who is this "I" that is constantly thinking and creating stress? You may reply, "Oh! It's me." Really?

Let's take a look at this "I". Can you show me where is it? It's in your head, isn't it? It's an abstraction, an illusion, a phantom. It is a *virtual* entity in your head that *steals* your identity. It is not the "true" you at all. Why do I say that? Because you are not born with this. In order to know your "True, Original Self," observe little babies, just a day or so old. I had the opportunity to be in charge of a well-baby nursery in my early career as a doctor and observed about sixty newborn babies every day. Later, I had the wonderful experience of having my own baby.

When you observe little babies, you see that as soon as their basic physical needs are met (i.e; a full stomach, a clean diaper and a warm blanket), they are *joyful* from within! They *smile* and go to sleep. They have no *past* or *future*. They are *not* worried if mom will be around for the next feed. If they did, they wouldn't be able to go to sleep. They don't think. Hence, there are no concepts, no judging, no anger, no *worries*. That's why they have no problem going to sleep. They are so *vulnerable*, but *fear* remains miles away. There is a total *lack of control,* but *no fear* whatsoever.

Once their stomach is full, they *don't* want any more food. If you were to force more food than they need, they would regurgitate. They eat to satisfy their hunger and that's all. *Wanting more* does not exist and that's why they are so *content.* You could feed them breast milk, cow's milk or formula. To them, it doesn't matter as long as it agrees with their stomach and satisfies their hunger.

They don't say "I don't like your milk, Mom. I like formula milk better." You won't hear, "Mom, you wrapped me in a pink blanket with butterflies on it. I'm a boy. Therefore, I need a blue blanket with pictures of dinosaurs on it."

They are joyful just looking around. They truly *live in the moment.* They do it *spontaneously* without making an effort to live in the Now.

Why do I say newborn babies don't think? Because, you always think in terms of a language. Newborns know *no* language. Hence, we can conclude babies don't think. They also have no concepts. Why? Because concepts arise out of language. No language - no concepts.

Newborn babies don't like or dislike someone because of their color, religion, nationality or wealth. That's because they have *not* acquired any *concepts* about religion, nationality, history or money. *Concepts* do not exist at all. *Likes and dislikes* do not exist. There are no *preferences or judgments.* No *embarrassment or shame.*

*No anger, no hate, no wanting more, no prejudices, no fear... Just pure joy, contentment and peace. This is the True Human Nature.* I like to call it the "True Self," the self that you and I and everyone else on the planet is born with.

Now let's see what happens to this fearless, joyful and peaceful baby.

## The Acquired Self

Gradually, another self develops as you grow up in a society. This, we can call the *Acquired Self*. You *acquire* it as a result of *psychosocial conditioning*, from your parents, your school and then, your society in general.

As you grow, this Acquired Self gets bigger and bigger. It gets in the driver seat, pushing the True Self onto the passenger side and later, into the back seat and eventually, into the trunk.

As a grown up, all you see is this Acquired Self. You identify with this Acquired Self. *That's who you think you are.* **This becomes the virtual "I" sitting in your head.** Your identity gets *hijacked* by the Acquired Self. Instead of seeing the hijacker for what it is, you think that's who you are. How ironic!

*This Acquired Self is the basis for all of your stress. It reacts to outside triggers, which it calls stressors and blames them for your stress. In fact, it is the Acquired Self who reacts to triggers and creates stress for you. In this way, the real source of all stress actually resides insides you. It is good to know this very basic fact. Why? Because if the source of stress is inside you, so is the solution.*

This Acquired Self torments you and creates stress even when there is no stressful situation. It conveniently creates *hypothetical* situations (the What If Syndrome) to make you fearful. I like to call it a *monster*, as it is quite frightening and appears strong, but in the end, it is really virtual.

Sadly, you don't even have a clue what's going on, because you completely identify with the Acquired Self, the *mastermind* behind all of your stress. You could call it the *enemy within*.

Unfortunately, you're completely out of touch with your True Self, the source of true joy, contentment and inner peace. In the total grip of the monstrous Acquired Self, you suffer and suffer and create stress not only for yourself, but for others as well.

Where does the Acquired Self come from? It comes from psychosocial conditioning from your society as you grow up. In this way, your Acquired Self is the *offspring* of your society, which itself is a collective Acquired Self, we can call the Society's Collective Acquired Self.

Your Acquired Self starts with the virtual "I", which is actually a concept that gets downloaded into your head. Your parents carefully select a label for you. They call it your name, which is basically a sound. Your parents utter this sound as they point towards you. After doing it repeatedly, they finally succeed in drilling into your head that you are indeed Peter, Sarah, Ali or Rekha. At the same time, they also drill in the concepts of Mama and Dada.

As you grow up in a society, you acquire more and more concepts, which circle around the concept of "I," just like the layers of an onion.

## How Your Acquired Self Creates Stress For You

Once your Acquired Self *steals* your identity, it *runs* your life. Then, you experience life through the *filters* created by your Acquired Self. These filters come from concepts, knowledge, information and experiences. The experiences can be your own as well as the experiences of others (virtual experiences for you), in the form of stories and opinions you saw in newspapers, books, magazines, TV or the internet or heard from friends and family.

Basically, your Acquired Self wants to live a very secure life. It wants security. Why? Because it is *inherently* insecure. It is *not* real. It is virtual, a phantom, an illusion, but it thinks it is real and it wants to live forever. Pretty crazy, isn't it?

In order to be safe, your Acquired Self *interprets* every experience (real experience or virtual experience. It doesn't matter) based on the information stored in it and *judges* the experience to be good or bad, which triggers an emotion, good or bad. Then, it *stores* the entire experience along with the triggered emotion into your *memory* box, where it stays *alive*, even years later. This is how your Acquired Self creates your *memories* or the <u>past</u>. Based on the past, it creates some more thoughts, it calls "My Future."

## Stress Created by the "Past and Future"

By keeping the old *dead* events alive, your Acquired Self keeps the *fire* of old emotions burning inside you. It calls them "my past" and "my memories." It judges these memories as either good or bad.

By replaying bad memories, your Acquired Self continues to experience the *negative* emotions attached to these memories in the form of *humiliation, anger, hate, bitterness, jealousy and revenge.*

By replaying good memories, your Acquired Self starts to *miss* those wonderful experiences and becomes *sad*.

## Acquired Self Wants to Change Its Past

Here's another interesting phenomenon. The Acquired Self wants to control the virtual world of memories. It is strongly attached to sweet memories, but it wants to run away from bad memories Therefore, it tries to modify the stories and events.

*For example:*

*"If my teacher hadn't humiliated me in front of entire class, I'd be a happy person today."*

*"Why didn't I see the clues? He's been cheating on me all along! Why did I marry him?"*

*"Why did I take this job? My boss is so stingy and demanding."*

*"Why didn't I sell my stocks six months ago when the financial market was so high?"*

But of course, the Acquired Self can't change what has already happened. It feels *annoyed, frustrated, angry* and sometimes *guilty* as well. The more it tries to change those painful memories, the stronger they get. What an irony!.

## The Acquired Self Wants To Secure A Happy Future

In addition, the Acquired Self doesn't want any bad event to happen again, ever! It wants perfect *security*. Your Acquired Self has been conditioned to learn from the past. Therefore, it wants to create a perfect world for itself in which there are only good things, and bad things do not exist. It wants to create a paradise for itself. Therefore, it continues to generate new thoughts along the lines of how to prevent bad events from happening again.

## The "What If" Syndrome

But then another thought erupts: *"What if I can't prevent it from happening again?"* That triggers huge *fear and anxiety.*

Caught up in the "What if, What may, What will I do Syndrome," your Acquired Self creates a virtual movie. In this way, it creates a huge amount of *fear* in you. In the pursuit of security and peace, your Acquired Self *robs* you of any peace of mind you had. How counterproductive!

Some examples:

*"What if I lose my job again?"*

*"What if my boss insults me again?"*

*"What if I become fat again?"*

*"What if I lose it again?"*

*"What if I get stung by the bee again?!"*

*"What if my audience makes fun of me again?"*

*"What if I become poor again?"*

*"What if I lose my friends again?"*

*"What if I get dumped again?"*

*"What if I'm late again?"*

*"What if I miss my flight again?"*

*"What if no one pays attention to me again?"*

*"What if my husband cheats again?"*

*"What if I have an attack of asthma again?"*

<u>In reality, those situations don't exist at all</u>. In other words, your Acquired Self is so *insecure* and *afraid* of its own death, that it creates all *possible,* dreadful case scenarios and tries to *figure out* how it can *escape* its death in every possible way. In doing so, it creates tons of *unnecessary* fear for you.

## Acquired Self Creates Attachment And Avoidance

Experiences which are labeled good, your Acquired Self wants *more* of and the ones labeled bad, it wants to *run* away from. This is the basis of psychological *attachment* and *avoidance*.

Your Acquired Self gets very *attached* to good experiences, such as praise and validation, which provides a *temporary* relief from its insecurity. That's why your Acquired Self gets attached to the <u>concepts</u> of *money, power, success and beauty*, all of which bring it praise and validation and provides *temporary relief* from insecurity.

Your Acquired Self also gets *praise* from family, friends and fans regarding its success, fame and accomplishments. It wants more and more of these experiences. It also feels *validated* when it is related, bonded or responsible for someone.

For example, if you own a pet, it *validates* the existence of you as an owner and provides your Acquired Self a temporary relief from insecurity. That's why it doesn't want to ever *lose* its pets, family, friends and fans. *Even the idea of losing them rips through the paper thin layer of security and stirs up deep-seated, inherent insecurity which triggers a huge amount of fear.*

Your Acquired Self also seeks validation through conceptual identities such as a doctor, lawyer, teacher, political, social or religious leader, movie star, employee of a certain company, citizen of a certain country, member of a certain social, political or religious group, etc. That's why even the thought of losing its virtual identity creates a huge amount of fear. This is why you are so afraid of the possibility of losing your professional license, career, citizenship, elections, etc.

Your Acquired Self does not *ever* want to *lose* anything or anyone that is "Mine." That would mean losing a part of "Mine." How terrible that would be! That's why it is afraid of losing possessions. The more possessions you have as "My, Mine," the more you *fear* losing them and the more you try to protect them. You may end up living in a gated community to protect your belongings. Even news of someone getting robbed creates a lot of fear for you.

In addition, your Acquired Self wants to *avoid* unpleasant experiences, such as failure, punishment, loneliness, humiliation, poverty, aging, disease and death at all costs. *Even the thought of such unpleasant experiences triggers intense fear.*

## Acquired Self Interprets Every Situation/Person

Your Acquired Self also quickly wants to *interpret* every situation it encounters and every person it meets, based upon *stored* information. Why? Because it wants to feel secure. It quickly judges if a person is safe or unsafe, based upon their appearance, without even exchanging a word. Judging triggers emotion. For example if it judges a person to be unsafe, you will start to experience fear, even though the other person has not done anything to you.

Often, it doesn't want to take any chances, so it won't interact with anyone it doesn't know. You may remember "don't talk to strangers" from your childhood. You also want to make sure to download this very important message into the growing Acquired Self of your children. Maybe you read a story about some girl who got abducted by a stranger in a far away place you know nothing about. It rips through your feeling of security. Ironically, it reinforces your self-fulfilling prophecy of being "fearful of strangers." Obviously, you don't hear or pay attention to the countless safe encounters with strangers.

## Acquired Self Creates Expectations

Your Acquired Self is downloaded with the concept of "how others should and shouldn't behave towards you and how you should and shouldn't behave towards them." For example, you expect certain kinds of behavior from your spouse, parents, brothers, sisters, friends and colleagues and *vice versa*. In a way, society dictates how each of us should fulfill our role. We can call it the *book of role descriptions*, written by the Collective Acquired Self of Society. Each and every person living in a particular society is downloaded with this *book of role descriptions*.

Everyone knows the description of his/her role and also knows the description of the role of others. For example, this book tells you *how a wife should behave, how a husband should behave, how a parent should behave, how a friend should behave, how a child should behave, how a teacher should behave, how a doctor should behave, etc.* Automatically it gives rise to certain expectations.

You *expect* others to play their part right, by the book. They *expect* you to play your role right. Now what happens if someone doesn't play their part right? You get frustrated and at times, angry. It's actually your Acquired Self who feels let down, frustrated and angry, because it is the Acquired Self who builds up expectations. Your Acquired Self believes in all of the concepts contained in the book of role descriptions.

The closer the relationship, the higher the expectations... And more emotional pain if someone does not meet your expectations. This emotional pain manifests as annoyances, frustrations and anger.

Examples:

- *A spouse falling off the ladder of expectations is the most frequent cause of divorce. It goes something like this: In a marriage, as soon as the period of intense sexual romance has cooled, the deeper layers of two Acquired Selves show their faces. Now each spouse starts seeing faults in the other person as the person is not living up to expectations. This initially causes annoyance which continues to build up in the memory box and eventually leads to pain and anger. Then one day, there is a big blow up and the marriage ends up in a divorce.*

- *Brothers, sisters and close friends get mad and angry if their expectations are not met. Sometimes they end up losing lifelong relationships.*

- *Kids failing to meet the expectations of their parents cause a lot of pain and suffering for their parents as well as themselves. For example, parents expected their son to become a doctor, but the son got poor grades in school. This caused severe headaches and ugly arguments between the son and his parents.*

- *Parents expected their daughter to marry someone they thought suitable for her, but she married someone else. Another cause for anger and pain.*

- *A wife expected a gift on her birthday but didn't get anything. The result? Hurt, pain and anger.*

- *A husband expected his wife to be nice to his rowdy buddies, but she called them immature dirt bags which caused a huge argument, pain and anger.*

- *An employee expected a raise, but didn't get one which caused pain and resentment.*

- *A person expected wonderful golden years after retirement, but ended up having cancer which resulted in bitterness and anger, in addition to the pain of the news of cancer.*

- *In addition to their own personal life, people also build expectations around political and religious figures, movie stars, singers, artists, etc. and get very disappointed and angry if their icon doesn't live up to their expectations. Some even get so angry that they end up killing their icon.*

- *People also create expectations around political, economic and religious systems and get very upset once their expectations are not fulfilled.*

- *People even have expectations about "how long they will live." It is called **life-expectancy**. We feel cheated if someone close to us dies before they were supposed to.*

The Collective Acquired Self of Society promises you that you will be rewarded if you follow the rules and punished if you don't. Now what happens if you follow the rules and don't get rewarded and someone who doesn't follow the rules gets rewarded? You get very upset and angry.

For example, you are an honest person suffering economic hardships while some crooked, dishonest liar is rolling in money. "Life isn't fair" you may find yourself saying. You feel very disappointed and angry at life.

## Acquired Self Creates Self-Righteousness

Another common reason for anger and frustration is self-righteousness.

What is self-righteousness? In simple terms, it means "I am right." It also *implies* that "you are wrong." This is the root cause of all disagreements, disputes, arguments, quarrels, fights, lawsuits, battles and wars, all of which obviously create a huge amount of anger.

With few exceptions, everyone suffers from self-righteousness. Interestingly, people don't like to be called self-righteous because it's considered a bad quality. They don't think they are self-righteous, but they readily see it in others. They simply judge others to be self-righteous and don't go any deeper. Actually, they believe they are *right* that someone else is self-righteous. Interesting, isn't it?

Self-righteousness is an extremely common affliction and one of the reasons for all human conflicts. If we want to understand human conflicts, it makes sense to look at self-righteousness more deeply.

## What is the Basis of Self-Righteousness?

Why do we believe that we are right and others are wrong? For example, for the same event, different people will have different opinions. Each one believes that he is right and others are wrong. The event is the same, but its interpretations are very different. Obviously, the problem lies in the interpretations. Now who is it that is doing the interpretation? It's your Acquired Self, isn't it?

Typically when a person looks at an event, his Acquired Self *interprets* that event against the background of the already stored information in his conditioned mind. Obviously, this stored information varies from person to person. Therefore, interpretation of the same event varies from person to person. A majority of people are in the grip of their Acquired Selves. Therefore, they strongly believe that their interpretation of the event is *right*.

If we look deeper at the composition of a person's Acquired Self, we find that the *book of role descriptions* is an important part of it. This book, as we observed earlier, describes how a person *should* and *should not* behave in a given society. In addition to creating expectations, it also provides a background against which everyone keeps *judging* others' behavior. It tells you and everyone else "what is *right* and what is *wrong*"; "what is *virtue* and what is *evil*." This is the basis of *morality*.

In addition to the *book of role descriptions*, your Society also downloads into your Acquired Self, many other concepts. For example, it gives you the concepts about "your rights," "human rights," "animal rights," "traffic rules," "sports rules." All of these concepts become part of your Acquired Self and give you more ammunition to be *right*. These concepts strengthen your self-righteousness.

When you are in the grip of your Acquired Self, these concepts and rules become your *beliefs*. When others don't follow the rules, you get frustrated and angry. For example, you are on the road, following the traffic rules and some other driver does not. Your Acquired Self judges you to be right and the other person to be wrong. This makes you furious. This is the basis of road rage, which sometimes, can lead to physical violence.

In addition, your Society downloads into your Acquired Self the knowledge of history, which primarily is an interpretation of certain events by the Acquired Self of the historian-writer. That is the reason why there are so many different interpretations of the same events and of course, every historian believes he is right. The historian's interpretation of events becomes part of your Acquired Self and you believe them to be absolutely true (although the event may have happened before you and the historian were even born). Different Acquired Selves with different versions of the same historic event or historic figure then get into heated arguments and get angry at each other.

With this background, your Acquired Self also judges current political, social and cultural events. Usually, it is some so called expert who does it for you, on a TV show, in a newspaper or in a book. Acquired Selves with different versions of history interpret current events differently and each one believes he is right. With this background, people get into heated arguments and get mad and angry at each other.

It is interesting to note that in a given society, there are collective concepts about what is right and what is wrong. This creates a *collective self-righteousness*, which gets reinforced constantly by the news-media in that society. *What is right in one society may be wrong in another society.* This creates conflict between various societies. That's why people living in one society get angry at another society. This is the basis of *collective conflict, anger and violence* between various nations.

Then, within a given society, there are various concepts about what is right and what is wrong, depending upon various social, political and religious groups in that society. This creates conflict, anger and violence between various groups within a society.

Then within a group, there are various concepts about what is right and what is wrong. Therefore, within the same group, people get angry and fight among each other. Even within a family, there are various concepts about what is right and what is wrong. It leads to conflict, anger and violence (usually verbal but sometimes even physical) between various members of the same family. For example, your husband may believe in disciplining the kids and you don't. This could lead to a serious argument and verbal conflict.

Then, within an individual, there are conflicting concepts of what is right and what is wrong. There is one code of ethics for the work place and another one for home, one code of ethics for friends and another one for enemies, one standard for yourself and another one for everyone else.

It all boils down to "I." Based on the concepts attached to your virtual "I," (your Acquired Self), you judge everyone else out there as either your friend or enemy. That's how you perceive other people - as either your friends or your enemies: at home, in your neighborhood, at your work place, in your social, political or religious group, in your country and in the world. You stay annoyed and angry at your enemies, which often leads to violence, verbal as well as physical.

### Acquired Self Reacts To Insults

Another reason why people get angry is *insults.* Obviously, you get angry when someone insults you. You *may or may not* express your anger.

Many people fight back by returning insulting remarks or gestures. Also, there are those who *pretend* to be polite and civilized on the surface, while fuming with anger underneath. Later, they often express their anger while talking to their spouse or friends. Some even suppress anger so deeply that on the surface, they *manage* to remain polite and civilized all the time. They may even try to *fake* a smile, but deep inside, they feel irritated and don't even know why they feel that way!

## What is the Basis of Insults?

Is it possible for you to *never* be insulted? I'm not talking about suppressing your anger and pretending that you are not insulted, but in reality - to not actually feel insulted at all when someone insults you.

In order to be truly free of insults, you first need to figure out, "who is it inside you who gets insulted in the first place."

Use logic and you will find that it's your Acquired Self who gets insulted. *The True Self never gets insulted.* Why do I say that? Because a newborn baby never gets insulted. *You can try to insult a baby by saying whatever you want, but the baby will not be insulted.* In the same way, imagine some one trying to insult you in a language or through gestures that you don't understand. Obviously, you will *not* be insulted. Therefore, we can conclude that for the insult to occur, one has to understand the *concepts* attached to those words and gestures. Otherwise, they have no power.

Where do you learn the words and gestures and all of the concepts attached to them? You are not born with them. You obviously learn them as you grow up in a certain society. That's why it is logical to conclude it's your Acquired Self who gets insulted.

With every word, there is a concept attached. For example, the word STUPID has a whole concept of unintelligence, inadequacy and worthlessness attached to it. When your developing Acquired Self learns this word, it stores all the negative concepts attached to the word. When someone calls you that word, the negative concept attached to that word is activated and negative thoughts trigger negative emotions. You feel unintelligent, worthless and inadequate, which triggers anger. *You didn't deserve it. How dare someone say that to you.* Actually, your Acquired Self's sense of self-esteem is threatened. Therefore, your Acquired Self fights back verbally or even physically in order to secure its existence, its self-esteem.

The insulting words are created by the Society Collective Acquired Self for the individual Acquired Selves to fight with each other, aren't they?

Society's Collective Acquired Self downloads the concept of *"insult and respect"* into your Acquired Self. When others respect you, your Acquired Self feels validated and when others insult you, your Acquired Self feels humiliated. In other words, your Acquired Self is constantly *reacting* to how others treat it.

Your Acquired Self wants to be respected and not be insulted. Obviously, it has no control over others' behavior, but it doesn't know this basic fact. It just keep searching for respect and running away from insult. It is especially true if at an early age, you were insulted (teased) a lot. Your Acquired Self felt humiliated and all of those painful experiences become part of your Acquired Self. Then, your Acquired Self found a way (academics, sports, arts, etc.) for others to start respecting you. Your Acquired Self finally got the praise and validation it was so hungry for. Naturally, your Acquired Self works hard on this track and usually ends up being quite accomplished and successful in that field. With each step of success, it gets more respect, praise and validation and it loves it all. *The more it gets attached to respect, the more it resents the idea of insult.* Then, a trivial teasing remark can upset your Acquired Self for days. You may even burst into anger in a social situation where you didn't get enough respect, which you perceive as an insult.

## Your Acquired Self Gets In Competition And Comparison

During psycho-social conditioning, *competition and comparison* are drilled into the developing Acquired Self. You see it everywhere: at home, at work, at school, at parties, on TV and practically in every walk of life.

## How Competition Creates Stress For You

When you're in competition, you either win or lose. What happens when you win? You get praise, validation and recognition. For that moment, you're the king of the hill. You have this wonderful feeling – a natural high filled with thrill and excitement. A few moments later, it's gone. You want more of it, but the moment, the occasion has passed. Now you have to work hard to be the "king of the hill" again. It takes a lot of hard work to be the champion, the winner, the outstanding person again.

The more victories you have, the more *addicted* you become to the momentary thrill and excitement. There is no ending. You simply want more and more and keep working in that pursuit. This is how you become greedy.

A competitive mind never gets enough and therefore, is always dissatisfied. You may be a wealthy, powerful, accomplished person, but inside you are empty, unhappy and dissatisfied.

Dissatisfaction leads to more greed for momentary pleasures and that means you must earn more money, fame, recognition, etc. It's a *vicious* cycle which often leads to various addictions, such as addiction to work, power, career, etc. You have *no* time for your family. Consequences: unhappy spouse, unhappy kids and often *divorce* which causes more emotional pain.

## How Comparison Creates Stress For You

Comparison lies at the root of ego. *"I am better than the others because of so and so."* The Society's Collective Acquired Self provides you with plenty of reasons to feel better than others. These ego-maker concepts include wealth, success, fame, knowledge, culture, genealogy, heritage, possessions, looks, appearances, religious, political and social clubs, etc.

Locked in the prison of ego, you feel quite miserable. On the surface, you're accomplished, famous and successful, but deep inside you feel empty, jealous and irritated. When society makes you feel *special* by acknowledging your success, your heroic actions or your special talents, you get a momentary thrill and excitement, but then it *fades* away... And you want more. You are never satisfied. You can't get enough praise, validation or recognition. You always want more.

Society of course, can't provide you with praise and recognition all the time. Often, it starts criticizing you as well. *First it builds you up and then it brings you down.* Then you feel miserable. You want others, especially your close friends and family members, to like you for your accomplishments and achievements. Instead, they generally stop liking you because they don't approve of the way you act under the influence of your ego.

An egocentric person is in the total grip of his own Acquired Self. He interacts with the world from the *virtual* castle of his own grandiosity. Why and how is this castle of grandiosity built? The Acquired Self builds this virtual castle in the pursuit of emotional security. It wants to suppress the fire of insecurity and worthlessness. It wants to be someone that everyone praises, validates and acknowledges instead of mocking, humiliating or criticizing.

For example, as a child or as a teenager you were subjected to comparison or criticism by some authority figure, such as your mother or your teacher. You felt the pain of humiliation and worthlessness. You also probably felt that you didn't deserve it. They were simply being *mean* to you. These thoughts of meanness and unfairness provoked intense anger inside you. All of these thoughts and emotions were stored in your memory as a constant nagging voice of criticism.

*You may or may not be aware of these humiliating experiences any more.* Some of these experiences, especially from early childhood, may have been forgotten. However, in your subconscious mind, these experiences are very much alive.

From these humiliating experiences comes another inner thought, "I'll never be humiliated again" or "I'll prove them wrong!" This inner thought becomes your *drive* to succeed in the world. It makes you work hard. You accomplish a lot, become successful and earn a lot of money and respect.

You get strongly attached to "success," as it validates you and provide a momentary band-aid on the old, but very much alive, wound of humiliation and anger. Attached to your success, you develop a *big* ego. On the surface you are accomplished and successful, but inside you still feel worthless, humiliated, irritated, angry and dissatisfied.

Then, a little thing triggers your inner anger to the surface. You are easily annoyed and have outbursts of anger over things that wouldn't bother other people - things such as someone *not* agreeing with you or making an innocent, unflattering remark. Why does this trigger your anger? Because you expect them to acknowledge and validate your success. When they don't, you feel like they are *criticizing* you and you over-react with all your piled up anger. This behavior causes you to lose some true friends. You want validation from your friends, but your actions push away your true friends. How ironic!

You keep proving to others and yourself over and over again how great you are, but it's never enough to heal your inner wound of worthlessness, unfairness and anger.

Actually, the more successful you become, the bigger your ego becomes and the more easily you get angry over little things.

Some people may not have gone through (or may not remember) humiliating experiences. However, they (their Acquired Self) learn from the Society's Collective Acquired Self that success, money, power or connections with powerful people are very important to live a "successful life" and they start to believe in this delusion. You (your Acquired Self) get praise and validation through your success, accomplishments, money, power, possessions, looks, etc. Each time it gets validated, its inner insecurity temporarily subsides, so it feels thrilled and excited. Unfortunately, all of this vanishes quickly and then it wants more... And the circus goes on!

*Ego* can take another form that most people are unaware of. Many people get attached to failures, losses and misery, either due to their own experiences (losses in competition and comparison) or collective losses of their collective identity (such as a religious, cultural or political groups). Then they (their Acquired Self) feel *special* in being a failure or miserable... the famous "Martyr Syndrome."

## Acquired Self Leaves You With *No* Time

People often complain they have *no* time. They are so busy with their life that they have *no* time to relax, *no* time to go for a walk, *no* time to prepare their meals......

Have you ever looked at where your time goes? Look at your activities during the day time *objectively* and you will find out where you end up spending your time.

In the grip of your Acquired Self, most people want to make more and more money. In the pursuit of "making more money" you end up working day and night, which is often full of demands and challenges. A lot of individuals also *commit* to a number of social obligations, which are also demanding and time-consuming. However, in the end, there is a reward, recognition or praise, which your Acquired Self is so hungry for. Therefore, you continue to work day and night and carry on your social obligations as well.

Then, you suffer from the "No Time Syndrome." You find yourself on the run. You stay rushed, agitated and restless. You don't have any time to prepare your meals. You grab a quick breakfast, often cereal, as you don't have any time to cook your meal. You may even drive through a restaurant to grab your meal and eat it inside your car while driving. Often, you have to travel a lot. Then, you may end up grabbing your meal at the airport, which is often unhealthy fast food.

Another reason people don't have any time is their *addiction* to "entertainment" in one form or another. Even after a long day, people come home and turn on their TV or go straight to their computers for entertainment. It is actually a great escape that your Society's Collective Acquired Self teaches you in order to *decompress* from the stress of daily living, which is, in fact, created by Society's Collective Acquired Self. Interesting, isn't it?!

At some point during entertainment activities, you may suddenly realize it's time for dinner. Then, you think of something you can prepare fast: a frozen dinner, a pizza, hot dogs etc, that you can throw in the microwave, while you go back to your *screen* of entertainment.

Chit-chatting is another common black-hole of time. Watch how much time you spend chit-chatting face-to-face, on the phone, internet, etc.

As a result of a "rat-race for money," social obligations, entertainment activities and chit-chatting, you are left with *no time* to prepare your meals, eat your food in peace or go for a walk. You are always in a rush. This is one of the main reasons why your blood sugars stay high.

## Acquired Self Keeps You Trapped In Partying

Most people get off their diet and indulge in unhealthy eating behavior during parties. Under social pressure, you *cave in* and end up eating a large amount of food, which is often unhealthy stuff.

Why do you end up *sabotaging* your good eating habits? Pay attention and you will see you lose all control of your eating when you are in a party. It's as if some inner *monster* takes over and lures you into eating all sorts of unhealthy foods. This is your Acquired Self, isn't it?

Starting from a young age, your Society's Collective Acquired Self downloads into your personal Acquired Self, a long list of *special* days that *must* be celebrated with food, often very unhealthy food. Birthdays, religious and national holidays and anniversaries are some examples. In addition, there are many other opportunities for celebrations. In general, the more successful you are, the more parties you go to and the more you end up eating unhealthy food.

All parties are *centered* around unhealthy foods and often, a large amount of food. Parties are also a lot of fun. In this way, Society's Collective Acquired Self downloads the concept of "food and fun" into your growing Acquired Self, since early childhood. You stay in this *mental* prison for the rest of your life.

After partying, you see your blood sugars as well as your weight going up. You don't like it. You feel like a big failure. You also feel *guilty* for cheating on your diet. Once again, you promise yourself that you will do better in the future and stay *disciplined* on your diet, which you are able to do until the next round of parties and you fall off the wagon again.

## Acquired Self Creates All Of Your Stress

It is pretty clear that your Acquired Self creates all of your stress. The Virtual "I," sitting at the core of your Acquired Self, looks at life through the *filters* of concepts, ideas, rules, information, past and future, which triggers a burden of emotional stress. Emotions then taint your thoughts. Emotional thoughts trigger more emotional distress.

A *vicious* cycle of thought-emotion-thought sets in. This is the basis of worrying, anxiety, anger, frustrations, hate, revenge, jealousy, guilt, thrill, excitement, greed, agitation, restlessness, sadness, and depression. Then, actions arise out of emotional thoughts which often cause more stress for yourself and others. The actions may be verbal, written or physical.

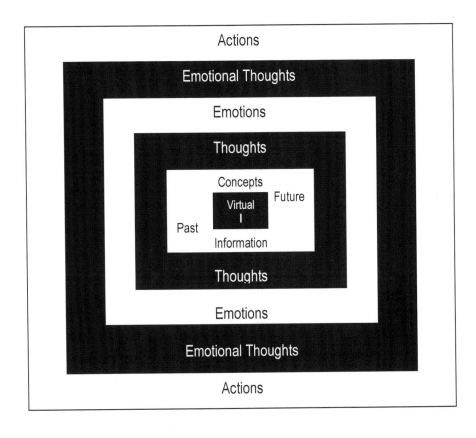

The Acquired Self

# How The Acquired Self Raises Your Blood Sugars

As we just observed, your Acquired Self makes you indulge in *unhealthy eating behavior*, which is the main reason your blood sugars keep escalating.

In addition, there are other mechanisms for how your Acquired Self raises your blood sugars.

The Acquired Self triggers emotions: anger, frustrations, annoyances, anxiety, jealousy, excitement, thrills, restlessness, agitation, sadness, and depression. Each of these emotions is *harmful* for your overall health, especially for those with diabetes. How do emotions affect your blood sugars? This is how.

Anger, frustrations, annoyances, jealousy, excitement, thrills, restlessness, and agitation cause an increase in your *adrenaline* level. Adrenaline is a hormone from your adrenal glands, which in turn causes an increase in your blood sugar levels. In addition, adrenaline also raises your blood pressure and can cause an acute heart attack or stroke.

Worrying, anxiety, and panic attacks also cause an increase in your *adrenaline* level and raise your blood sugars. In addition, these emotions raise *cortisol*, another hormone from your adrenal glands. Cortisol causes further increase in your blood sugar by worsening your insulin resistance.

Sadness and depression cause an increase in your *cortisol* level, which subsequently raises your blood sugars. Sadness often leads to "emotional eating behavior." You end up eating all sorts of comfort foods which are laden with sugar, carbohydrates and fats. Naturally, your blood sugars go through the roof after eating those kind of foods.

In addition to raising your blood sugars, your elevated cortisol also wreaks *havoc* on your immune system.

## How To Be Free Of Your Acquired Self

The Acquired Self is obviously the root cause of all of your emotional stress and its harmful effects on your diabetes as well as your overall health. The obvious question is: How can I be free of my Acquired Self?

A word of caution: Don't try to *control* or *discipline* your Acquired Self. This strategy simply *strengthens* your Acquired Self and creates more stress. Also, do not start to dislike/hate your Acquired Self. This creates a *negative* attachment, which further strengthens the grip of your Acquired Self on you.

See your Acquired Self for what it is. In fact, the Acquired Self is a *tool* to function in society. It's only when it steals your identity - you mistakenly think that's who you are - that it gets in the driver's seat, takes control of your thoughts, emotions and actions and creates emotional stress for you.

Therefore, you need to rise above your Acquired Self. Then, you can utilize it as a tool to function in society and put it to rest when it is not needed.

First of all, you have to see your Acquired Self as *separate* from you. Only then, can you see it for what it is. However, if you continue to *identify* with your Acquired Self, you can *never* see its true colors. As long as you and your Acquired Self are *stuck* together, obviously you can *never* be free of it.

In order to *free* yourself from your Acquired Self, you have to see it in action. When you're in the grip of your Acquired Self, you *immediately* react to *triggers*. We can call it <u>auto-pilot</u> mode. These automatic reactions often cause more stress for you and others. Later on, when you come to your senses, you often *regret* what you said or did.

## 1. Pause!

The *first step* to *separate* yourself from your Acquired Self is to *not* let it automatically control your actions. Pause! Stop for a moment, before you *react* to what you heard, read or watched.

## 2. Shift Your Awareness/Attention To The Now

Shift your attention to the *Now*. What is Now? Now is *not* what is in your head, but what is in front of your eyes. It is your <u>field of awareness</u>.

Pause for a moment right now and pay attention to what you see, what you hear, what you smell, what you taste and what you touch. Don't think, just sense.

In general, when we see, we only pay attention to objects without paying any attention to the *space* in which everything is.

Without space, there would be no objects. So when you see objects, also be aware of the space which gives rise to all objects. Also when you see some movement, be aware of *stillness* in the background. In the same way, when you listen, also pay attention to the *silence*, without which there would be no sound.

Use your eyes and ears and be aware of 3-S': *space, stillness, silence,* which gives rise to all objects, events and sounds.

In addition to your outer field of awareness, you also have an *inner field of awareness.* This inner field of awareness is your *Original, True, Self.*

It is vibrant, full of immense energy, joy and inner peace. No words can accurately describe it... But it can be felt. It is Real and not a concept. That's why your Acquired Self, which consists of concepts, cannot understand it. You can feel your inner field of awareness simply by taking your attention inside your chest.

In fact, your outer field of awareness is an extension of your inner field of awareness. It is <u>one</u> field of awareness... And that is what the Now is! I made this *arbitrary* distinction of inner and outer field of awareness just to communicate with you. That's all!

Practice to be aware of the Now around you and inside you. Then, you can easily *shift* your attention to the *Now* as soon as you realize your thoughts and emotions have taken you over.

The moment you switch your attention to the Now, you are free of your thoughts and their associated emotions. In other words, you are free of your Acquired Self. *Instantaneously,* you will feel *relief* from anger, fear or any other stressful emotion. That's how powerful this seemingly simple step is. A moment later, your attention may again be *sucked* up by the thoughts and emotions. It's okay. Simply keep shifting your attention/awareness into the Now.

Your Acquired Self needs your *attention* to thrive. That's why it *sucks* up your attention/awareness most of the time. However, you have the power to *switch* gears and *divert* your attention/awareness to the Now. Without your attention/awareness, your Acquired Self can *no* longer survive. As long as your attention/awareness is in the Now, you are *free* of the Acquired Self.

Remember this phrase: *Keep your mind where your body is.*

While fully aware of the Now, feel and watch the drama your Acquired Self creates. Don't run away from it. After a little while, it will settle down.

Example:

You're stuck in traffic on your way to the airport. You start worrying. "What if I miss my flight?" Then you may blame your spouse ,"If only you had listened to me and left on time, we wouldn't be in this mess. You *never* listen to me anyway." Your spouse *fires* back with some *ugly* words that triggers more anger inside you. Engaged in a verbal fight, you both get upset and angry. Then, you may see some driver *not* following the traffic rules. You may *yell* at him and experience road rage. You may get so angry from the drama that your Acquired Self creates, that you may end up having chest pain and find yourself heading to a hospital... Or you can choose to shift your attention from thoughts to the Now: Watch the car in front of you, the cars to each side, the median of the freeway, the electric poles seemingly running backwards, the sky, the clouds, etc. Also pay attention to your breathing, which is a *continuous* act in the Now.

Chances are pretty good that you will arrive at the airport safely, certainly without any anger or high blood pressure or high blood sugar. You may or may not be late. If you are late, you will deal with it.

Therefore, live in the Now, stay in reality and you won't have any emotional distress.

<u>Caution:</u>

Be careful *not* to confuse *attention* with *concentration*. Attention is simple awareness, that's all! It is there automatically, without any effort. On the other hand, concentration and discipline require a lot of effort and are quite stressful by themselves.

## 3. Use Logic - Common Sense

Now take the next step: use *logic*, the most wonderful tool we humans have. Why? Because the Acquired Self is always *illogical* and can't stand the blazing *torch* of logic. Therefore, use logic and see the *true colors* of your Acquired Self. See for yourself who is really at the root of all of stress. See how *illogical* your Acquired Self is.

For example, you *fume* over things that happened in the past: Someone *insulted* you, *betrayed* you, *let you down,* etc. Use logic and see for yourself that no matter how much you think about your past, you can *never* change it. "But I must learn from it so it must *never* happen to me again," says an inner voice. With that kind of mind set, what people often end up learning is *mistrust, jealousy, hate and revenge.* They also become *fearful* that it may happen again. In fact, you keep your past *alive* (although it has otherwise *died*) as long as you stay in the mind set to *learn* from it. Only when you completely *let go* of your past, you can be *free* of the emotional trauma it caused you.

Emotional pain from the past also comes in another form: *sweet memories.* Even thinking about all the good times makes you *sad.* In fact, the more you think about "sweet memories," the *sadder* you get. Use logic and realize those "sweet memories" are nothing more than an *illusion,* a *dream,* a *phantom.* Those events were "Real" when they happened, but now they are simply a package of *mental pictures, stories* and associated *emotions.* Only when you completely *let go* of your "sweet memories," can you be *free* of sadness caused by them.

Another example: Your Acquired Self may be worried about its future. Use common sense and you'll see whatever your thoughts imply may or may not happen... But certainly, it's not happening in the Now, in front of your eyes, right? Therefore, it's a phantom, an illusion. How can you really take care of a problem that doesn't even exist? If and when it happens, at "that time, the present moment," you'll be able to take *real* action, instead of the *virtual* action your Acquired Self keeps thinking about, which serves no purpose, but simply generates fear.

Another example: You are in your sixties and doing fine. Then one day, you read in the newspaper that someone important died of cancer. Your Acquired Self triggers a thought... What if I have cancer? This creates another thought of possibly losing your health, autonomy and ultimately dying. This creates a huge amount of fear. You start to feel your heart pounding. You feel uneasiness and anxiety. Then, you start wondering who'll take care of your wife if you die, which further worsens your fear and suddenly, you've got a full-fledged panic attack.

Even in the *midst* of this panic attack, pause, take some deep breaths and start counting your breaths. Look around and see what is actually happening in front of you. Feel the space inside your chest. At the same time, feel the fear, but don't get consumed by it. Fully realize that it is your Acquired Self who is fearful. Your True Self, is untouchable. Then, use logic. Ask yourself: Do I have cancer at this moment? Am I losing my autonomy at this moment? You realize you really don't have any problems at this moment. Then, you also clearly see that it is actually your Acquired Self playing tricks with you by creating an imaginary future. The moment you clearly see the Acquired Self for what it is, an entity separate from you, it starts to lose its power over you. Using logic, you also tell your mind: "I will deal with any medical condition, if and when it arises." Make a mental note to discuss it with your doctor on your next visit or even write it down on a piece of paper. You will see fear completely evaporate and you can move on with your everyday life.

In addition, *acknowledge* the basic law of nature: if you are born, then one day you die. There are *no* exceptions to this rule. The Acquired Self however, does not want to die and wishes to live forever. Therefore, it makes death something you must avoid, cheat, conquer, etc. In this way, it creates a lot of *negativity* about death. In the grip of their Acquired Self, many people *worry* about death all their life and then one day they die. How sad!

Stop worrying and start living. You can do it once you are free of your Acquired Self.

Instead of worrying, take action in the present moment. For example, eat right, exercise regularly and take vitamin D every day. There's a good chance you won't develop cancer, heart disease or Alzheimer's dementia, etc. Even if you do develop any medical condition, you will be able to deal with it at that time.

However, if you just keep worrying and don't take any actions, chances are you may develop these diseases. Take real action in the present moment, instead of worrying about the results.

Next time you find yourself saying," I don't know where all of my time goes. I feel so *pushed* all the time." Use logic and look at all of your activities, engagements and commitments, from a *neutral* ground. Then, figure out what are important activities for basic living and what are the activities for ego-enhancement, thrill, excitement and entertainment.

Next time you are in a party, realize your body has not changed because you are in a party. Eat to satisfy your hunger, not to *appease* your friends and family members.

Use logic and realize special days are special, because Society's Collective Acquired Self says so. In Reality, they are just another day in Nature.

Caution:

Please be aware that I am using the word logic as the simple common sense that every human is born with. I am not using it as intellectualization, rationalization or reasoning.

---

## 4. Be Aware Of The Conceptual World We Live In

Have you ever pondered about the world we live in? If you take a fresh, logical look at the human world without preconceived notions, you will find that we live in a *conceptual world*, a *virtual world*, not a real world.

Because everyone around us lives in this collective conceptual, virtual world, we think it is real. Actually, we simply accept it as real and don't even bother investigating whether it is real or not.

For example, let's say you watch the Oscar Awards on TV. Through the goggles of the conditioned mind, (your Acquired Self), you see five actresses nominated for best actress. After a few moments of agony, everyone is told who wins *best actress of the year*. The winner is obviously thrilled and excited, but the other four feel defeated, though they try to force a fake smile. For the winner, the moment has finally arrived, the moment for which she has waited for years. She gets overwhelmed with emotions, but manages to deliver an tearful speech. Then, her moment is over. In a few minutes, it is someone else going through similar emotions.

If you are a serious moviegoer, you have your own opinion as to *"who deserves to be the best actress."* If your choice wins, you are also *thrilled*, but if your choice loses, you will be *disappointed*, sometimes even *angry* and *bitter* about the *unfairness*.

You and the world calls it *entertainment*. You want more of it and the world is well-equipped to provide you with more! Over the next several days, you enjoy seeing more and more about the whole event on the internet, TV, newspapers and magazines. You see stories about before and after parties, designer dresses, behind the scenes, etc.

For the next few days, you even talk to your friends about the whole experience and have more fun. Actually, the more you know, the more you can impress your friends and the more special you feel about yourself.

Now, let's look at the whole event from an <u>unconditioned mind - someone without the Acquired Self</u>. Now, what you see is a person coming on stage to receive a shiny peace of metal. Holding that piece of metal in her hands, she gets very emotional, her eyes become tearful and her voice chokes. She says a few words and then everyone starts clapping. Why, you wonder?

Obviously, that piece of metal has a huge *concept* attached to it. The woman appearing on stage is not just a woman, but has a huge *concept* attached to her. The whole drama has a huge *concept* attached to it. *The entire concept reverberates with the concept in your head and in everyone else's head, about Oscars, actresses and actors, movies and the concepts of success, achievement, fame, wealth and glamour.*

In other words, your Acquired Self, the *Baby* Monster, gets fed by the *Papa* Monster of the society! That's why you enjoy it so much. For you and everyone else, it becomes real. Actually, you don't even question whether it is real or not. You watch and talk about it as if it was real.

*It is interesting to know that you may be able to see the superficial, virtual nature of the part of the conceptual world that you are not attached to.* For example, if you are attached to sports and not to movies, you may *not* be interested in watching the Oscars and may even realize their superficial nature, but you will *not* miss the Super Bowl, Wimbledon, the World Cup, the Olympics, etc. Each one of these words has huge concepts attached to them - the concepts of *victory, achievement, fame, wealth and glamour.*

If you use logic, you will find that most sports are about a ball that is kicked, thrown, carried and/or hit. The world does *not* see it that way. It sees these sports as a matter of *competition, victory, achievement, fame, glamour and wealth.*

By now, you may understand the virtual, conceptual nature of these events. However, you may say these are occasional events in your life. Well, take a close look at the usual activities of your daily life and you realize that most human activities are in the *domain* of the conceptual, virtual world.

Here are some examples: (*Let me make it very clear that I am making these observations using simple logic. I am not criticizing, putting down or making fun of any of these concepts. Of course, you don't have to agree with me.*)

The Internet, TV, newspapers and magazines obviously take you into the virtual, conceptual world. Many people start their day reading a newspaper or watching a morning show on TV. They glance through magazines or surf the internet during the day. In the evening, they usually watch TV or surf the internet. Most are hooked on TV or the internet for hours every day.

It's interesting to see some older people complain about young people wasting too much time on the internet, playing video games or texting. Meanwhile, they waste their time reading newspapers, watching TV and talking about politics or religion.

Everything you read in newspapers, magazines and books or watch on TV and the internet is conceptual and virtual, isn't it?

Everything in movies, stage shows, museums and art galleries is conceptual, isn't it? All pictures, paintings and statues are obviously conceptual.

All knowledge, whether history, mathematics, science, arts, geography or business is virtual and conceptual, isn't it? In this way, all of the educational system is conceptual.

Language itself is conceptual. Observe how every word carries a concept with it as we observed earlier in the book.

How about political and social systems? All are conceptual.

How about religious establishments? Those are all conceptual as well.

How about cultures, traditions and values? Those are all conceptual.

In reality, you see mountains, land, buildings, roads, trees, animals, sky, clouds and water. However, on a map you see continents, countries, states, provinces and cities - all conceptual.

How about marriage, romance, engagement, divorce? All are concepts, aren't they?

How about time? Seconds, minutes, hours, days, weeks, months and years. All conceptual. Different cultures have created different calendars.

How about national, religious and cultural holidays? All conceptual.

There are concepts attached to gold, platinum, jewels and diamonds. In fact, these are simply metals and rocks, but there are huge concepts attached to them.

How about money? This concept is so overwhelming that no one ever thinks of it as conceptual.

The Concept Of Money

Almost everyone is in the grip of the concept of money and the economy. For most people, it also creates a lot of worries.

What is the economy? It's a concept isn't it? You can not see the economy. You see currency, which itself is a concept. One Dollar, ten Euros, five Yen, a hundred pesos, fifty Rupees, etc.

If you give a 100 dollar bill to a one year old kid, she will probably put it in her mouth, chew on it or rip it apart. Why? Because she still has *not* acquired the concept of money. However, give the same 100 dollar bill to her when she is a teenager and she will be thrilled to have it. Why? Because by now she has acquired the concept of money. In reality, it is a piece of paper, but of course, there is a concept attached to it.

Everyone wants to make money. Money itself is a concept, but people don't think of it that way. To them money is real. *"You can't do anything without money,"* you may argue, but that still does not make it real. *It may be necessary to some extent, but it is not real. To live in the conceptual world, you need money, but it still does not make it real.*

If you look deeper, you'll find that money is a way for humans to *trade* with each other. Not too long ago, people also used chickens, eggs, rice, etc. to purchase services from each other.

Animals don't do any trading. Obviously, humans developed the *concept of trading.* The concept of trading came into being when humans started living in communities. For example, "I can exchange my eggs for your wheat." Initially, it served a purpose, but then it took over the human race. The concept of precious metals and money came into being. The more money (or precious metals) they had, the more they could buy. Initially, they bought things of necessity: food items, clothes, houses...

But this was not enough. They wanted to acquire more and more. Why? Because society also created other concepts: The concepts of prestige, fame, glamour, enjoyment, entertainment, vacations and power. The more money you have, the more powerful, the more famous and the more prestigious you are. You can also have a high profile life-style.

With money, you can purchase various conceptual objects: the car of your dreams, your dream home, your dream vacation, etc. Money is *no* longer just a means to buy the things of basic necessities. It is often used to *enhance* your ego, which is part of the Acquired Self.

These days, "wanting more" is the driving force behind the concept of money. There is never enough of it when you are in the grip of "wanting more." Even a *billionaire* wants to get more!

## What's Wrong With Concepts?

There is nothing *inherently* wrong with concepts. It is only when they are not treated as concepts, but as reality, that they become *problematic* and create stress for you and others.

Use logic and you'll realize that *concepts are not reality and reality is not conceptual...* But all humanity is lost in concepts and believes in them as if they were absolute truth. People get attached to concepts. They either love them (positive attachment) or hate them (negative attachment). Then, actions arise out of these attachments. Actions arising out of concepts create a huge amount of stress for you as well as everyone else.

Concepts also divide humans into groups. Each group believes their own concepts to be true. This obviously creates *conflict*. One group sees the other group as a *threat* to their collective belief system, which creates collective fear. This often leads to violence, verbal as well as physical and can even lead to battles and wars.

## 5. Utilize Your Acquired Self To Function In The World

The collective *conceptual* world, which we call the world, downloads a *conceptual* world into everyone's head, which is their Acquired Self. The two worlds are *extensions* of each other and *feed* each other. Basically, it is one big *conceptual* world.

Do Not start to hate your Acquired Self. In fact, your Acquired Self has its relative significance. It is your tool to function in the conceptual world, but obviously it is *not* you. The problem arises when you mistakenly believe your Acquired Self *is* you and you lose your true identity. Then, you are enslaved by your Acquired Self, which creates tons of stress for you and others. On the other hand, you need to *rise* above it and be its master, not its slave.

While interacting in the conceptual world, utilize your Acquired Self, but don't get overtaken by it. As soon as you don't need the assistance of your Acquired Self, switch gears and shift your attention to the Now.

## 6. Stress Free Living

With few exceptions, everyone is consumed by the *conceptual* world in their head, their Acquired Self and the collective, *conceptual* world, which we call the <u>world</u>.

As we observed, the conceptual world is full of stress. That's why people are so stressed out. They don't see any way out. They often *rationalize* their stressful living with statements such as "Oh, stress is part of life. There's nothing you can do about it." Then, they seek refuge in *escapes,* such as drugs, alcohol, partying, vacationing, gambling, etc, which provide only temporary relief and actually add more stress in the long run.

Once you *clearly* realize the *conceptual* nature of the "I" and the *conceptual* nature of the world, you are *free* of them. With this *mental* shift, a profound wisdom sinks in and your life becomes *stress free* automatically.

For example, you realize <u>money is a concept.</u> It helps you earn a living in the conceptual world, that's all! You earn money to meet the basic *necessities* of life such as food, shelter, clothing, transportation, etc. However, you clearly see the difference between "necessities" and "wanting." You realize it is the Acquired Self that has a never-ending list of "wanting," which is the basis of greed and lack of contentment.

You also clearly see how the Acquired Self *boosts* up its ego by pursuing certain respectable professions, by seeking fame, by living in a mansion, by acquiring certain possessions or by living a certain lifestyle. You also see the rat-race everyone is in to make more and more money and how it creates a huge amount of stress in their life.

Once you are free of wanting, greed and ego, you are *content* with whatever job or business you are in, as long as it provides you with the income to make a basic living.

Once you are *not* in the rat-race any longer, you have plenty of time to prepare your meals. You can actually sit down and enjoy your meal.

When you are not attached to your house, possessions or lifestyle, you are not worried about losing them.

Once you are free of your ego, the need for praise and validation evaporates. The emotional drama of respect and insults comes to an end.

In the grip of the conceptual world, a lot of people end up doing shady stuff to make more money. Then, they are *afraid* of being caught. Once you are free of greed, you obviously don't get into illegal practices to make more money. Then, you're *not* afraid of being caught, because you're not doing any shady stuff.

In addition, you don't seek your *identity* through your profession, certain title or position. Then, you *don't* have thoughts about losing them and worries remains miles away.

As a student or parent of a student, you are no longer in a race to go to a prestigious university. As a student, you figure out what you're good at and pursue that particular field. It may or may not bring you a lot of money, but you are fine with this, because you are free of your Acquired Self and therefore, free of wanting, greed and ego. In this way, you don't have to go through tremendous worries such as "What if I don't get accepted at a prestigious university?"

You realize rules are concepts, but you also acknowledge their functional value. Therefore, you *follow* traffic rules, you *follow* campus rules, you *pay* your income tax and you *follow* the rules of your profession or business. In this way, you become a perfect law-abiding citizen. You have *nothing* to hide. Then, you have *no* fear of being caught.

Once you realize all rules are concepts, you follow them yourself, but don't judge others if they don't. In this way, you don't fume over "those bad people" who don't follow the rules on the freeways, in offices, in political, religious and cultural parties etc.

Once you realize *expectations* and *morality* arise out of the "book of role descriptions" written by your society (how everyone should and shouldn't behave), you automatically stop having expectations. Consequently, you have no disappointments, annoyances and anger.

In addition, you automatically stop judging all of "those immoral, bad people." You do your role by the book, but don't judge others. In this way, you stay free of a lot of frustrations and anger.

You realize political systems and parties are conceptual. Then, you don't get into heated arguments with others over political issues. Your don't get angry watching TV shows or reading newspapers. You realize you can *impact* your virtual political system by casting your vote every few years and that's all. You don't keep fuming over elections results when your party doesn't win.

You realize marriage is a concept, but you also realize its functional value and *follow* it as a part of living in a society. Free of your Acquired Self, you don't get into the mess of extra-marital affairs, which is the activity of the Acquired Self to enhance its ego or to escape from emotional pains. Obviously, if you don't have any affairs, you don't worry about being caught.

You realize beauty is a concept. Consequently, you *don't* worry if you lose a few hairs, if your hair start turning grey or if a wrinkle or a pimple appears on your face. You don't need to dye your hair, apply wrinkle cream or see a plastic surgeon. All the *worries* about side-effects of these dyes and creams, the high cost of plastic surgery and its possible side-effects automatically do not arise.

You recognize the conceptual nature of all sports, television shows and the stock market. Then, you *don't* worry about the loss of your team, the fate of your favorite TV show or the performance of your stocks.

You realize that internet, TV, newspapers and magazines keep you *trapped* in the conceptual world. Automatically, you don't spend much time on these activities. Then, you don't hear sensational, horrifying and dreadful news and stay free of unnecessary fear.

You realize "special days" do not exist in the Real world, but only in the conceptual world. Then, you don't have *expectations* from others to do certain things on certain special days, such as birthdays, anniversaries, religious and national holidays. No expectations means no disappointments if someone does not live up to your expectations. You also become free of self-criticism and guilt.

You realize your life, in Reality, is a line between birth and death. It is your society's Collective Acquired Self that *artificially* divides this line into *segments* such as childhood, youth, middle age and old age. Then you are free of *anguish* once you turn forty.

Once you clearly see the virtual nature of the past and the future, you don't *fume* over painful memories or *miss* the good old times or *worry* about the future. You also become free of the collective emotional pains of your group, race or nation, due to history being kept alive. At the same time, you don't worry about the collective future of your group, race, nation or the entire human race. Instead, you keep your attention in the Now - what is in front of you, what you sense with your *five* senses.

Once you realize that concepts divide humans into political, social, cultural and religious groups and create conflict, you automatically are not *emotionally* attached to them. In this way, you become free of the collective "hate and revenge" that *plagues* the majority of the human world.

Once you realize the universal law of birth and death, you don't worry about death. In order to deal with a disease, you take the appropriate medicine and make necessary changes in your diet and exercise level. *You realize you are alive until the moment you die.* <u>You realize life is to live and *not* to worry.</u>

In short, you *minimize* your interactions in the conceptual world to the bare <u>necessities</u>. In this way, you *free* up a lot of time to spend in the Real world, the Now, where there are no worries, frustrations, anger, regrets, hate, jealousy, sadness or worthlessness. And it is *not* a boring life. Quite the opposite!

Once you are in touch with your True Self, you tap into an *immense* source of joy and inner peace. Then, you have no need to seek thrill, excitement and entertainment.

That's how you live a life that is *joyful*, *peaceful* and completely *free* of the emotional stress.

*To learn more about stress management, please refer to my book, "Stress Cure Now."*

Chapter **11**

# My New, Scientific Approach To Diabetic Diet

Proper nutrition is the most important step towards taking charge of your diabetes. Most diabetics know this basic fact. However, they continue to struggle with their diet. They feel frustrated. Many get demoralized. There are several reasons why your diet does not work for you and why you don't stay on your diet. Perhaps, you'll see various aspects of your own struggle with your diet as we proceed through this chapter.

## Why Most Diets Fail

I'm sure you've resolved many a time to change your diet in order to avoid the horrible diabetic complications your doctor keeps talking about. For a few days or even weeks, you follow your diet diligently. However, eventually you slip up or slack off or give up. Slowly, you gain back all the weight you lost. You're back to square one. Do you ever wonder what really happened? You want to do what's good for your health, but you end up doing what's bad for your health. Crazy, isn't it?

Take heart: diabetics aren't by any means the only category of people who struggle with this issue. Almost everyone sometimes feels as if there's someone else controlling their mind. Most people hear that inner voice that says, "Oh, that wonderful cake. A little piece won't harm me. Life is short, enjoy it." If you obey this inner voice, before you know it, you've finished that piece of cake.

Unfortunately, if you've had trouble sticking to your diet and/or are presently overweight—whether you are diabetic or not—it's likely that this inner voice is largely in control of your eating behavior! It enslaves you. So before you can make any true, everlasting change in your eating pattern, you need to be free from this inner voice. Before you can be free of it, you need to fully understand it. This inner voice comes from your Acquired Self, as I elaborated in the previous chapter.

The inner voice that keeps you off track and off your diet consists of memories, concepts, and ideas that swirl around in your mind. From your childhood, you learn that pleasure and fun comes from food. Birthday parties, holidays, family get-togethers—at each occasion, food is the center of the celebration.

You're encouraged to overeat. Often, this food is unhealthy. Cakes, pies, cookies, donuts, pizza: the list goes on and on. Yet it's all wrapped up in the warm glow of fun and pleasure. As you grow up, you keep adding memories of fun and pleasure through overeating . This is how your mind gets conditioned and then controls your eating behavior. Your inner voice comes from your conditioned mind.

The collective food associations in your particular society or culture play an important role in conditioning your mind. How many times have mothers implored their child to finish the food on their plate because children are starving in other countries? You are told you need to grow up to be big and strong. In many societies, this association holds true, especially for males. The bigger you are, the stronger you are. Sports heroes are often big guys.

The more you can eat, the more macho you are. Restaurants offer buffet deals: eat as much as you want for the same price. Eating contests reward the winner who eats the most. Restaurants brag about the size of their servings—the biggest hamburger in town, etc.

In the workplace, snacking is commonplace. I'm amazed at the amount of food I see at the nurses' station in the hospital.

My techie friends tell me they usually have a bag of chips and a can of soda when they're at the computer. Even at physicians' conferences, just after we've had a talk about the epidemic of obesity and diabetes, we take a break for a snack filled with donuts, pastries, and soda.

Often food is an expression of love, respect, and gratitude. Mothers might show their love, for instance, by baking chocolate-chip cookies and apple pies. As a grown-up, you'll have a hard time resisting them. Frequently, you may not be hungry, but you eat to please or be respectful to others. Friends may actually get their feelings hurt if you don't eat their food.

Your buddies may badger you to drink a beer with them while watching a football game. Food is more like an emotional bond between parents and children, between friends and colleagues, and between people of the same culture, geographic location, or religion. If you dare not participate, you're an outcast. Can you even imagine not eating that wonderful Thanksgiving dinner or refusing all those Christmas treats? We all want to blend in, be part of our food-celebrating culture, even if it means damaging our own health.

You were having such a wonderful life, full of parties and food for pleasure, and then one day, diabetes ruined it all. Suddenly, you're told to change everything you've been doing your whole life. Your inner voice says, "No way! I'm not going to give up all the fun that comes from food"

Your inner voice - your conditioned mind - your Acquired Self controls your eating behavior. This is the main reason you don't adhere to a good eating pattern for more than a few days. You're up against a lifetime of pleasurable, unhealthy, conditioned eating behavior.

So, how do you get freedom from this understandably powerful inner voice? You do it with logic and awareness.

Use logic. Eat only when you are hungry: not for fun, not for pleasure, not to stuff down your depression. Eat because you are hungry and your body needs food.

Be aware of your actions. Often people are not fully aware of their actions and stay on auto-pilot mode. For example, they grab a bag of popcorn while watching a movie or they keep drinking soda while working on a computer. Office workers keep snacking on crackers, cookies and candies that someone brought to the office. You go to the grocery store and automatically pick up a carton of ice-cream, soda, bagels, etc.

Pay attention to your actions. Only then you will be able to see how *illogical* your actions can be. Then, you will be able to stop these illogical automated actions.

For example, in the grocery store, pay full attention to every item that you buy. Use logic: Do you need this food? How is it going to impact your diabetes and overall health? With awareness and logic, you will obviously buy only those foods that are healthy for you.

Each time you are tempted to indulge—whether at a party, or when you're feeling sad and lonely—pause, shift your attention to the Now (your surroundings), let your emotions settle down before you take any actions. Use simple logic and your true intelligence that helps to pierce through the treacherous layers of your Acquired Self.

See for yourself that all of the so-called special days - birthdays, anniversaries, religious and national holidays - are in fact, conceptual in nature. Each special day has a concept attached to it: how it should be celebrated. Your metabolism does *not* change on these special occasions. Wake up and see for yourself that we live in the conceptual, virtual world created by the collective human mind most of the time.

Instead of being lost in the virtual world in your head and your thoughts, shift your attention into the reality of the Now: What you see, hear, smell, taste and touch. Also, be aware of the 3 S' - space, silence and stillness. Take attention into your chest. Feel the *inner peace* and *joy* you are born with. It is always there! You don't pay attention to it. That's why you don't feel it.

Once you get in touch with your true nature of inner peace and joy, you no longer chase emotional pleasures. You no longer run away from emotional pains. This is how you become free of all of the celebrations of the special days. This is how you become free of the addiction of food.

Don't turn your diet into some sort of discipline, which will make you feel like you are in a prison. Sooner or later, you want escape and break your disciplined eating pattern. Then, you may finish a half gallon of ice cream in one sitting. Shortly afterwards, you feel guilty and sad. Low self-esteem crawls in. "I don't have what it takes to stay disciplined. I'm a loser, so I may as well eat some more ice cream."

Who is generating sad thoughts? Your Acquired Self. Who is blaming? Your Acquired Self. Isn't it interesting to observe that your Acquired Self got you into a bad eating pattern in the first place. Then, it tells you to *discipline* your eating habits. Then, it generates thoughts that trigger emotions of failure, sadness and guilt.

Just remember, your Acquired Self is not the true you, as you were not born with this destructive behavior. You acquired it from society due to  psycho-social conditioning as you grew up.

Awareness of your actions, instead of discipline of your actions, is the key difference between your True self and your Acquired Self. Be aware of the Now, be aware of your hunger, be aware of the food items, be aware of the quantity of food, be aware of your satiety, be aware of tempting, illogical emotional thoughts.....

With awareness and simple logic, you can be free of your age-old, unhealthy, conditioned patterns of eating.

Now, let me share with you my own awakening as an endocrinologist about the "Diabetic Diet."

# My Own Awakening About Diabetic Diet

Back in my early days as an endocrinologist, I used to send my diabetic patients to dietitians. In addition, I would buy booklets on diabetic diets from our big medical organizations and give them to my diabetic patients. These diets were developed by the most prestigious dietitians, and were based on Calories, typically an 1800 calorie diet. Then there were 1600, 1400, and 1200 Calorie diets. But nothing was working. My diabetic patients continued to have high blood sugars and I continued to keep adding more drugs to control their diabetes.

I got frustrated with my diabetic patients for *not* following the diet, until one day this very nice old lady replied gently, "but I am following the diet you gave me and my diabetes is still out of control." I could see the truth in her eyes. She was referring to the diet booklet I had given her on her previous visit. Suddenly, a thought popped into my head that would drastically change my outlook about diet: "What if the diabetic diet itself was incorrect?!"

As a true scientist, I wanted to find out the truth myself. So I decided to use myself as a guinea pig. I calculated the number of calories I needed per day, using the standard formula I had learned during my medical training. Then, I used the recommended formula to figure out how many grams of carbohydrates, protein and fat I needed per day. I put myself on the "healthy" diet, according to the scientific formulas which I used to believe in as the *gospel* truth.

To my utter surprise, I gained 5 Lbs. in a two week period. I was shocked. How could it be? I had not changed my exercise level. The only thing I changed was my diet and it caused me to gain significant weight in a short period of time.

## Calorie-Based Diet-Approach Is Unscientific

After the initial shock, I embarked on a journey to develop my own diet, starting from scratch, using logic as my guide. First of all, I realized the concept of calories was actually very *unscientific* when it comes to human health.

For a moment, let's set aside the *mantra* of calories that we all have been indoctrinated with. Let's us do some fresh scientific investigation. What is a calorie? It is a unit of heat energy, first described by a French chemist, Nicolas Clément in 1842. He was working with the amount of heat-energy produced from burning coal, in relation to powering steam engines. Later, the chemists started to use the concept of calories in terms of heat produced during chemical reactions in the laboratory. Then, this concept got into biochemistry. How many calories can you get from burning one gram of carbohydrate, fat or protein in a calorimeter, which is a device to calculate the amount of heat energy. Then, this concept was applied to food and the human body and that's where things went wrong. Why? Because food is much more than heat energy and the human body is much more than a calorimeter.

Food is *not* just calories, but it contains nutrients that provide nutrition to the body. Nutrition is much more than the heat energy or the calories. The highly prevalent concept of *calories in-calories out* is accurate in a laboratory, but it does not quite apply to the human body. Why? Because the human body is extremely complex. The function of a given cell depends on so many factors, such as genetics, hormones, vitamins, enzymes, coenzymes, blood supply, nerves input, chemicals from immune systems and the list goes on and on.

For example, you give the same amount of calories to two different people, the results on their weight, blood sugar and other health parameters will be quite different, even though these two people are of the same age and do the same amount of exercise. I have often heard my patients say, "But my friends consume more calories than me and I'm the one with the weight problem. It doesn't make any sense." Even the same number of calories from carbohydrates versus fat have a different impact on your weight, blood sugar and other health parameters.

Even how food is prepared has a huge impact on your health. For example, the same number of calories as juice versus whole fruit has an amazingly different effect on your blood sugar. Raw fruits and vegetables have a different impact on your blood sugar compared to cooked fruits and vegetable with the equivalent number of calories. Steamed foods have a different effect on your blood sugars compared to fried or grilled foods. The same amount of calories coming from olive oil versus margarine have different effects on your body.

Thinking of food simply in terms of calories has lead to the development of foods which are *low* in calories, but have no nutritious value and often have *horrendous* health consequences. Diet sodas are a good example. They contain little or no calories, but are loaded with chemicals, such as artificial sweeteners, sulfuric acid, nitric acid, and preservatives. All of these chemicals have a long list of health consequences: mental fogginess, jitteriness, indigestion, kidney damage, abdominal obesity, asthma, skin allergic rashes, dental decay, and serious damage to DNA.

People drink diet sodas under the impression that *less* calories means they will lose weight. Not true! In a study (1) from Purdue University, researchers found that diet soda drinkers were at increased risk of weight gain, Type 2 diabetes and cardiovascular disease.

### Diabetic-Diet Must Be Individualized

When it comes to diabetic-diet, it must be individualized. The one-size-fits-all approach is unscientific. Here are some facts to keep in mind:
• The appropriate diet for a *Type 1* diabetic patient is different from a *Type 2* diabetic patient.
• The appropriate diet for an obese person is different from that of a lean person.
• The appropriate diet for a seventy-year-old diabetic is different from that of a thirty-year-old patient. Our metabolism slows drastically as we age, especially after the age of fifty.
• The appropriate diet for a sedentary person is different from that of an active person.
• The appropriate diet for a diabetic patient taking pills is different from the diet of a diabetic on insulin injections. Diet will also vary depending upon the type of drugs you take.
• The appropriate diet of a *Type 2* diabetic on insulin injections is different from a *Type 1* diabetic on insulin injections.

- The appropriate diet for a diabetic on an insulin *pump* is different from a diabetic on insulin injections.

## My New, Scientific Approach To Diabetic Diet

Now you understand that here are many *variables* that determine the effect of a certain food on your blood sugar, such as genetics, age, your activity level and drugs that you are on. In this way, every person is *unique* and a certain food will have a *unique* effect on their blood sugar. Is there a way to put this cause-and-effect relationship between food and blood sugar into clinical practice? That would be very scientific, right!?

### CGM (Continuous Glucose Monitoring)

Fortunately, there is great clinical test, called CGM (Continuous Glucose Monitoring), in which a device smaller than a cell phone, is attached with a small plastic needle under your skin and it registers your blood sugar every hour for 72-hours. We utilize CGM in our *uncontrolled* diabetics, usually on their initial visit to figure out their *unique* pattern of blood sugars. Patients keep a food diary while they wear the CGM. The results are *shocking* for most patients. They can't believe that certain foods they thought were healthy (such as oatmeal and other healthy cereals), caused such a rise in their blood sugar level. It is truly an eye-opening experience for many diabetics.

### The Food-Sugar Diary

While CGM is a great test, it is somewhat costly and some patients' insurance company do not want to pay for it. In these patients, we assess the cause-and-effect relationship between food and blood sugar in another way. I advise my patients to check their blood sugar *two* hours after a meal and write it down in a diary, along with what they ate. You can call it a **food-sugar diary**. Ideally your blood sugar two hours after a meal should be less than 140 mg/dl.

Initially, you check blood sugar two hours after *every* meal. After one month, you pretty well know the cause-effect relationship of various foods on your blood sugars. Then, you can cut back how often you check your blood sugar, provided you are a Type 2 diabetic and *not* on insulin.

Obviously, you should consume those foods which keep your blood sugar under 140 mg/dl and avoid those that cause a sharp rise, such as a blood sugar more than 200 mg/dl. My patients bring their food-sugar diary on their visit and I review it with them.

CGM as well as The Food-Sugar Diary approach takes into account all of the variables in a particular food and your body that can affect your blood sugar. It gives you the direct result of the impact of a certain food on your body in terms of your blood sugar. It doesn't get any more scientific!

Based on this kind of sound clinical data over the past fifteen years in my diabetic patients, I have developed the following dietary recommendations.

Note:

As I mentioned earlier, there is no one diet that will work for every diabetic person. You have to carry out the cause-effect relationship between foods and blood sugars yourself, by checking your 2-hours post-meal blood sugars.

Use the following recommendations as a starting point.

# WHAT NOT TO EAT

### 1. No processed food.

No canned foods, snack bars, or pre-cooked dinners. Have fresh foods, real foods and organic foods. The true nutritional value of a food (compared to what is written on the food label) is lost when it is processed, stored or frozen.

Try to grow your own vegetables and fruits. In addition, use a local farmer's market to buy fruits and vegetables. Remember, if a fruit or vegetable has traveled hundreds, if not thousands of miles, it has lost its *true* nutritional value.

## 2. Reduce Starches And Sugar

Some common food items should only be used sparingly, because they are loaded with starches and sugar. These food items are:

- Bread, rice, pasta and pizza.
- Bread includes white bread, whole wheat bread, sourdough bread, French or Italian bread, bagels, croissants, biscuits, hamburger buns, rolls, pita, Indian naans, tortillas, tacos and many more similar bakery products.
- Cereals including oat-meal
- Potato chips, nachos, French fries.
- Waffles, pies, donuts, pancakes, pastries, cookies, candy, chocolate and cakes.
- Corn, potatoes, sweet potatoes, yams, barley and rye.
- Quinoa and some of the other "exotic, ancient" grains.
- Desserts, Ice-cream, Frozen Yogurt

## 3. Avoid Artificial Sweeteners

Avoid artificial sweeteners such as Sucralose (Splenda), Saccharin (SugarTwin, Sweet'N Low), Aspartame (Equal, NutraSweet), Acesulfame (Sunett, Sweet One) and Neotame.

Also beware of sugar alcohols such as Sorbitol, Mannitol, Xylitol, Lactitol, Maltitol, Erythritol, Isomalt, Hydrogenated starch hydrolysates (HSH).

These artificial sweeteners are widely used in processed foods, including sodas, powdered drink mixes, chocolate, cookies, cakes, chewing gum and candies. These products are typically marketed as sugar-free and low calorie, which obviously has great appeal to the general public.

As a general rule of thumb, stay away from all *processed* food items. These are NOT natural, regardless of what they claim. These are synthetic substances that may have started out from a natural substance, but the final product is far from anything that exists in nature. For example sucralose (in Splenda) is made when sugar is treated with trityl chloride, acetic anhydride, hydrogen chlorine, thionyl chloride and methanol in the presence of dimethylformamide, 4-methylmorpholine, toluene, methyl isobutyl ketone, acetic acid, benzyltriethlyammonium chloride and sodium methoxide, according to the book, "Sweet Deception." This processing obviously makes sucralose unlike anything found in nature.

Artificial sweeteners and sugar alcohols can give rise to a number of side-effects, including gas and abdominal cramping. Why? Because these chemicals are usually not absorbed properly and become a fuel for bacterial overgrowth in the intestines. Some even cause neurologic symptoms such as confusion, headaches or dizziness. In addition, there are serious concerns about their long term safety.

If you *absolutely* have to sweeten your food, you can use a small amount of honey. For example, 1/2 teaspoonful for your tea or coffee.

## 4. Avoid High Fructose Corn Syrup

Avoid any food that contains high fructose corn syrup. In fact, consumption of high fructose corn syrup can lead to obesity, diabetes, heart disease and liver damage.
High Fructose Corn Syrup also provides fuel for the growth of bacteria in the intestines and can cause bloating, cramping and excessive gas.

## 5. No Sodas, No Fruit Juices and No Alcohol.

Do not drink any sodas, even diet versions. Why? Because sodas are loaded with high fructose corn syrup and sugar. Diet sodas use artificial sweeteners and sugar alcohols.

Also avoid fruit juices, because fruit juices from grocery stores contain only a small amount of real juice and a lot of sugar water. Avoid even freshly squeezed, natural juice. Why? Because you end up consuming a high amount of natural sugar, fructose.

For example, instead of eating just one whole orange, you will have to use 3-4 oranges to get about a cup of pure orange juice.

Instead of fresh juice, eat one to two Fresh fruit servings per day. Why? Because whole fruits not only contain sugar (fructose), but also the pulp, which slows down the absorption of sugar. That's why there is less of a rise in blood sugar level after eating a whole fruit, as compared to fruit juice, which causes a rapid rise in blood sugar level.

Avoid alcoholic beverages. Why? Because alcohol is a medically well known toxin for the liver, pancreas, brain and nerves. In addition, alcoholic beverages contain carbohydrates and sugars. For example, most beer comes from malted cereal grains, most commonly malted barley and malted wheat.

## WHAT TO DRINK?

Water should be your beverage of choice. You can also use milk, tea and coffee in small amounts.

In a restaurant setting, order water for your drink. Many people order a soda in a restaurant under peer pressure. Remember your body has *not* changed because you are in a restaurant.

## WHAT TO EAT?

### 1. Vegetables

For clarification, when I use the term vegetables, I refer to the leaf and stem part of the plant, excluding the roots (such as potatoes, sweet potatoes and yam), which are basically starches.

Eat plenty of vegetables. Include vegetables in every meal. They are a great source of vitamins, minerals and fiber. They are bulk forming, fill up your stomach and satisfy your appetite. They also slow down the absorption of sugar from carbohydrates in your diet.

In general, vegetables contain only small amounts of carbohydrates, which is usually fiber. For example, 1/2 cup of cooked spinach contains only 3 gm of carbohydrates, out of which 2 gm is fiber. Spinach, like many other green leafy vegetables, is a great source of Vitamin A, Vitamin K and Manganese.

Use fresh vegetables of the season. Get them from your own vegetable garden or from a farmers' market. Try to steam them or lightly fry in olive oil.

Use raw vegetables in your salads, such as cucumber, bell pepper and tomatoes.

## 2. Fruits

Eat one to two fresh fruits or 1/2 cup per day. Always use fruits which are in season. Either get them from your own fruit trees or from a farmers' market. Avoid fruits and vegetables which have traveled all around the world.

There is tremendous wisdom why certain fruits and vegetables grow in a certain season and climate. We humans may never be able to comprehend this wisdom. Suffice it is to say that if you live *in sync* with nature, you will avoid a lot of health problems.

For example, nature produces summer fruits for people in a particular area who are also experiencing summer temperatures. Now, you may be in the winter season, but your grocery store is loaded with summer fruits, brought thousands of miles away from the other side of the equator. Without thinking, you grab these produce items as novelty items. Remember fruits and vegetables are just foods, not items for mental entertainment or ego enhancement.

Different fruits have a different impact on your blood sugar level. We can *categorize* fruits in terms of their potential to raise your blood sugars, according to our experience at the Jamila Diabetes & Endocrine Medical Center.

Fruits That Cause A Marked Increase In Blood Sugar. Therefore, consume them in very small amounts:

- Grapes
- Banana
- Watermelon
- Orange
- Mango

Fruits That Cause A Modest Increase In Blood Sugar. Therefore, consume them in small amounts:

- Apples, yellow
- Peach
- Plum
- Strawberries
- Honeydew
- Cantaloupe
- Figs

Fruits That Cause A Small Increase In Blood Sugar. Therefore, consume them in moderate amounts:

- Apples, green or red
- Blueberries
- Gooseberries
- Blackberries
- Raspberries
- Kiwi

A Few Words About Bananas

Often diabetics consume bananas under the impression that they provide Potassium. It is true that bananas are high in potassium, but they are also high in sugar. There are many other food items which are high in Potassium, but not high in sugar. For example, avocados are a great source of Potassium. In addition, avocados can help to increase your good (HDL) cholesterol, which is often low in diabetics. Avocados are also loaded with omega 3 fatty acids, vitamins C and E, carotenoids, selenium, zinc and phytosterols, which help to protect against heart disease and inflammation.

## Don't Stop Fruits Altogether

Some diabetics go to an extreme and stop fruits altogether. This *drastic* approach may help to decrease your blood sugar, but in the long term, it is *not* healthy. Why? Because fruits are a great source of vitamins, minerals and antioxidants.

As an antioxidant, they help to neutralize the damaging effects of free oxygen radicals that are released as a byproduct of the metabolism of food in the cell or when the body is exposed to cigarette smoking or radiation. These free oxygen radicals can damage the structures inside the cell. This is called *oxidative stress* and it may play a significant role in causing diseases such as cancer and heart disease. Anti-oxidants help to neutralize oxidative stress. Anti-oxidants consists of Beta-carotene, Vitamin A, Vitamin C, Vitamin E, Lutein, Lycopene and Selenium.

Brightly colored fruits are loaded with anti-oxidants. Fruits that are highest in antioxidant contents are pomegranates, blueberries, strawberries, cranberries, cherries, plums, oranges, and apples.

Fruits are also a good source of fiber, especially avocados, apples, pears, guavas, pomegranates, blueberries, blackberries, raspberries, oranges, figs and kiwi fruits.

## 3. Nuts/Seeds

Nuts and seeds are an excellent source of nutrition. They are a great source of Monounsaturated Fatty Acids (MUFA) and omega-3 polyunsaturated fatty acids. Together, these are called the good fats. Why? Because these fats help to increase good (HDL) cholesterol and lower bad (LDL) cholesterol.

Nuts are also a good source of protein, vitamin E (an anti-oxidant) and fiber. They are also low in terms of carbohydrates.

Nuts are also packed with vitamins and minerals such as magnesium, phosphorus, potassium, selenium, manganese, folate, copper, calcium and zinc. In addition, nuts contain phytosterols, such as flavonoids, proanthocyanidins and phenolic acids.

There is mounting evidence to show that nuts may reduce oxidative stress and inflammation. Clinical studies show that nuts can reduce the risk of heart disease, age-related brain dysfunction and diabetes (2,3).

Almonds, pine-nuts, pistachios and peanuts contain more protein than other nuts. Macadamias contains the highest amount of monounsaturated fatty acids, followed by hazelnuts, pecans, almonds, cashews, pistachios and Brazil nuts. Walnuts contain the highest amount of polyunsaturated fatty acids, followed by Brazil nuts, pecans, pine nuts, pistachios, peanuts, almonds and cashews.

Nuts also contain a small amount of saturated fat, the so called bad fat. Almonds contain the least amount of saturated fat and Brazil nuts the highest. While all nuts contain some selenium, Brazil nuts have the highest quantities. Selenium is a good antioxidant, helps the immune system and may prevent some cancers.

Pine nuts are one of the richest sources of manganese, which is an important co-factor for the anti-oxidant enzyme, superoxide dismutase. Consequently, pine nuts are good anti-oxidants. In addition, pine nuts contain the essential fatty acid pinolenic acid, which works as an appetite-suppressant by triggering the hunger suppressant enzymes, cholecystokinin and glucagon-like peptide-1 (GLP-1) in the small intestine.

Technically, peanuts are not actually nuts but legumes. Dry beans, peas and lentils are some other examples of legumes.

Like nuts, seeds are a good source of protein. For example, 100 grams of seeds will provide you with 30 grams of protein. Seeds are an excellent source of the amino acids tryptophan and glutamate. Tryptophan is converted into serotonin and niacin. Serotonin is an important regulator of our mood. Low serotonin can lead to depression. That's why many modern anti-depressant medications, such as Prozac, Zoloft, Paxil, Celexa and Lexapro act by increasing the level of serotonin in the brain. Glutamate is a precursor for the synthesis of γ-amino butyric acid (GABA), which is an anti-stress neurotransmitter in the brain and can help to reduce your anxiety.

Like nuts, seeds are also loaded with vitamins and minerals. Pumpkin seeds can block the action of an androgen, DHEA (Dehydroepi-androsterone). This may be helpful in preventing prostate and ovarian cancers.

Use raw nuts and seeds. Do not use salted, sugar-coated or chocolate-coated nuts or seeds for obvious reasons.

## 4. Meats/Poultry/Fish

Eat meats, poultry and fish, including shell fish. These are excellent sources of protein, vitamins, minerals and contain no carbohydrates. For example, 1 oz (28 grams) of cooked Atlantic salmon contains 6 grams of protein, 3 grams of fat, is loaded with Omega 3 fatty acids, and is also a good source of Thiamin, Niacin, Vitamin B6, Phosphorus, Vitamin B12 and Selenium (4).

Red meat is an excellent source of protein, iron and vitamins, especially vitamin B12. For example, 1 oz (28 grams) of ground Beef, (95% lean meat/5% fat, crumbles, cooked, pan-browned, hamburger) contains 8 grams of protein, 2 grams of fat, and No carbohydrates or sugar. It does contain 20 mg of cholesterol which is only 7% of the daily recommended value (5). Compare it to 1 oz (28 grams) of cooked Quinoa which contains only 1 gram of protein, 1 gram of fat and 6 grams of carbohydrates, but no cholesterol (6).

Eat red meat 2 - 3 times per week. Select lean cuts. Avoid processed meats such as cold cuts, salami and hot dogs, as these often contain added sugar and carbohydrates.

Eat Chicken and/or turkey once a day. These are great sources of protein and vitamins.

Eat Fish 1 - 2 times a week. In addition to providing you with protein and vitamins, these are great source of Omega-3 fatty acids, which are good for your cardiovascular health. However, overconsumption of fish can lead to mercury poisoning.

Remember, vitamin B12 is lacking in plants. Therefore, you often become low in vitamin B12 if you are on a vegan OR vegetarian diet.

## 5. Dairy

Eat a cup of regular, plain yogurt everyday. It is a great source of healthy bacteria for our intestinal health. It is also a good source of protein and calcium as well.

Include a moderate amount of cheeses in your diet. If you are trying to lose weight, then *limit* the use of cheese.

Drink a cup of milk per day, provided you are not Lactose Intolerant. If you have Lactose intolerance, you should try Almond milk.

A lot of individuals with lactose intolerance do well on yogurt and cheeses.

## 6. Eggs

Eggs are a great source of protein, vitamins and minerals, especially Riboflavin, Vitamin B12, Phosphorus and Selenium. Eggs contain no carbohydrates. Therefore, they are a great nutritional source for people with diabetes.

People are overly concerned about the cholesterol content of eggs. Cholesterol is present in the yolk of the egg. If your LDL cholesterol is elevated, then you should use only egg whites.

# HOW TO EAT

Eat three regular meals per day. Dinner should be the lightest meal of the day, lunch the heaviest and breakfast the modest meal. Eat dinner at least 3 hours before bedtime.

Avoid snacks, especially when you're watching TV or working on a computer. If you absolutely must have a snack, then try something like nuts, carrot sticks or other raw vegetables.

Get involved in your food. Read labels on food while you are in the grocery store. You'll be surprised how many food items contain sugar, fructose syrup and corn syrup. Avoid these food items.

Try to prepare your meal yourself, at least over the weekend. Avoid buffets! When you opt for a buffet meal, you want to get the most for your buck (after all, you're only human) and you generally end up overeating. Try to eat at home as much as possible. You can find my original recipes in Part 2 of this book.

If you are trying to lose weight, keep a diary of the food you eat. You may be amazed at how much you really eat, contrary to what you thought.

Eat when you are hungry, not because you're sad or on a computer or you have to socialize with family members and friends. *People often eat because of psycho-social reasons.* That's why they continue to gain weight.

Be aware of your eating habits. Eat slowly and enjoy every bite of your meal. Don't watch TV while eating. Many people overeat because they get too involved in watching a TV show or reading a newspaper and don't keep track of their food intake. Physically, you may be sitting at the dining table, but the TV or newspaper takes your mind hundreds and even thousands of miles away. When you're eating, your mind should be *aware* of what you're eating. Taste your meal, chew it properly, enjoy it. Observe other people sitting at the table and the ambience in the room. Relax! Take your time. Don't be in a hurry.

Read these recommendations frequently. This will serve as a reminder.

# Practical suggestions for meals

## Breakfast:

Egg omelet using 2-3 eggs. OR 2 hard boiled eggs.

OR

1/2 to 1 cup of yogurt. Add a handful of sliced almonds or blueberries or walnuts/pecans or cashews

## Lunch / Dinner:

A bowl of vegetable soup
A plate of grilled chicken and fresh garden salad (you may add salad dressing).
A fresh fruit such as a small apple
A handful of nuts (almonds, pistachios, walnuts/pecans, cashews.)

OR

A bowl of vegetable soup.
A small chicken or turkey or tuna in a lettuce wrap.
A fresh fruit such as a pear.
A handful of nuts (almonds, pistachios, walnuts/pecans, cashews.)

OR

Grilled vegetables such as bell pepper, zucchini or eggplant, with chicken or turkey strips, stir fried.
A handful of blueberries.
A handful of nuts (almonds, pistachios, walnuts/pecans, cashews.)

OR

Grilled Chicken or Steak.
Grilled or steamed vegetables.
A fresh fruit such as  a peach.
A handful of nuts (almonds, pistachios, walnuts/pecans, cashews.)

OR

Shrimp on a bed of steamed vegetables.
A fresh fruit such as half orange.
A handful of nuts (almonds, pistachios, walnuts/pecans, cashews.)

OR

A bowl of soup.
Fish, grilled or baked.
Few strawberries
A handful of nuts (almonds, pistachios, walnuts/pecans, cashews.)


# ETHNIC FOODS

## Chinese

A cup of won ton soup.
Beef or chicken or shrimp, cooked any Chinese style.
A fresh fruit such as a small apple

OR

Mongolian barbeque beef or chicken.
A fresh fruit such as half orange.

## Japanese

2-3 sushi. Avoid rice rolls.

Stir fried beef or chicken.
A fresh fruit such as a small apple.

## Mexican

A cup of vegetable soup.
A plate of chicken or beef fajitas, without rice or tortilla.
A fresh fruit such as a peach.

## Indian/ Pakistani

Two pieces of Tandoori chicken.
Mixed vegetables.
A fresh fruit such as a half a mango.

OR

Two Seekh Kebobs.
A plate of vegetables such as okra, spinach, or eggplant.
A fresh fruit such as a small apple.

OR

A small portion of chicken or beef or lamb curry, mixed with vegetables. For example, lamb saag or lamb okra or chicken jalfrezi.
A fresh fruit such as half orange.

## Middle Eastern

Chicken or beef kebob and salad.
A fresh fruit such as a handful of pomegranate seeds.

OR

Chicken shawarma.
Grilled vegetables.
A fresh fruit such half cup of melon.

## Greek

Greek salad.
Gyro meat (no fries or rice).
A fresh fruit such as a pear.


**Please see page 282 of the book for RECIPES**


**References:**

1. Swithers SE. Artificial sweeteners produce the counterintuitive effect of inducing metabolic derangements. *Trends Endocrinol Metab*. 2013 Sep;24(9):431-41

2. O'Neil, C.E., D.R. Keast, T.A. Nicklas, V.L. Fulgoni, 2011. Nut consumption is associated with decreased health risk factors for cardiovascular disease and metabolic syndrome in U.S. adults: NHANES 1999–2004. *Journal of the American College of Nutrition*. 30(6):502–510.

3. Carey, A.N., S.M. Poulose, B. Shukitt-Hale, 2012. The beneficial effects of tree nuts on the aging brain. *Nutrition and Aging*. 1:55–67. DOI 10.3233/NUA-2012-0007.

4.http://nutritiondata.self.com/facts/finfish-and-shellfish-products/4259/2

5. http://nutritiondata.self.com/facts/beef-products/6192/2

6.http://nutritiondata.self.com/facts/cereal-grains-and-pasta/10352/

Chapter **12**

# Exercise:

# How Much And What Type?

Exercise is one of the five-steps that helps you manage your diabetes. However, by itself, it is not enough. In addition to exercise, you have to pay attention to the other four steps, especially stress management and proper nutrition.

You should consult your physician before beginning an exercise plan. If you have heart disease or suspect you may have heart disease, check with your cardiologist before starting an exercise program. As a general rule, exercise should be started at a low level. Duration and intensity should be increased gradually.

### Excessive Exercise Can Be Harmful

We all know that lack of exercise is unhealthy. How about intense rigorous exercise? In my professional opinion, excessive **exercise** can be harmful as well, for the following reasons:

### 1. Excess Oxidative Stress

You are probably familiar with the term, "anti-oxidants." What are anti-oxidants? These are nutrients that help to fight off oxidative stress. What is oxidative stress? As a by-product of metabolism of food, oxygen free radicals (also called oxygen reactive species) are released inside the cell. These oxygen free radicals are toxic for the cell itself. This is what oxidative stress is. An analogy would be a factory, using coal for heat production.

In addition to heat, the factory also generates smoke and other toxic gases, which are harmful for the people working in the factory as well as the rest of the planet.

Now consider this. Intense exercise revs up your metabolism. Consequently, you have excessive amounts of oxidative stress. Your factory (your cell) is in high gear producing energy. Excessive smoke in the form of oxidative stress is the natural consequence. Excessive oxidative stress due to intense exercise is very *harmful* for your body, although you may feel *elated* during this type of exercise, which is due to the release of chemicals, such as excess adrenaline and endorphins.

## 2. Exercise-induced injuries

Intense exercise also predisposes you to all sorts of injuries: neck sprain, leg sprain, and tennis elbow are some examples.

In addition, excessive use of joints, over a period of time, contributes to degenerative arthritis, which then leads to chronic pain as well as limited activity level. Consequently, your insulin resistance and diabetes worsens. Remember, your diabetes is likely to get worse with time and you are going to need your legs, especially in your golden years.

**How Much And What Type of Exercise?**

I make the following recommendations about exercise to my Type 2 diabetic patients:

- Don't sit in front of a screen (computer or TV) for hours. Take frequent, few-minutes breaks and walk. During this time, also pay attention to your physical surroundings, without thinking. This will make you aware of the Now, in which there is no stress. Freedom from stress and exercise work together to lower your insulin resistance and blood sugar level.

- Do some stretches in the morning and in the evening. Simple yoga can be very helpful in this regard. Certain yoga postures can actually help to prevent as well as treat arthritis-pain.

- After stretching, walk for about 20-30 minutes in the morning before breakfast, as well as in the evening before and after dinner, on a daily basis.

- The morning walk helps you lower your insulin resistance and blood sugar due to the Dawn-Phenomenon. What is the Dawn-Phenomenon? In the early morning hours, your body produces large amounts of these hormones: *growth hormone, adrenaline and cortisol.* All of these hormones worsen your insulin resistance. Consequently, your blood sugar rises even before you have breakfast. This is called the Dawn-Phenomenon. Getting up early in the morning and going for a walk after doing some yoga is the best way to counter the effects of the Dawn-Phenomenon.

- The evening walks helps you to prevent acid-reflux in your stomach. In addition, it lowers your blood sugar the next morning.

- Swimming is a good alternative for those who have difficulty walking.

- Many diabetics have peripheral neuropathy in their feet. These patients should *definitely* avoid jogging or running, as it will worsen their peripheral neuropathy.

- Diabetic patients with retinopathy should *definitely* avoid jogging as it can be harmful to their eyes.

- Exercise can lower blood glucose too much, especially if you are on drugs such as Insulin, Prandin, Starlix or sulfonylurea drugs (such as Glucotrol, Amaryl, Glynase, Glipizide, Glyburide). Therefore, always carry candy while on a walk.

- Check your blood sugar before exercising. If your blood sugar is below 100 mg/dl, eat something before you exercise. Also check your blood sugar at the end of exercise.

- Actos (pioglitazone), and Metformin do not cause low blood sugar by themselves.

## Why Most People Do Not Exercise On A Regular Basis

Most people do not exercise on a regular basis because they do not have time for it. Why don't they have any time for exercise? Because they are caught up in activities of daily life. They keep planning to exercise: One day, once they have enough time, they will start to exercise. Obviously, that day never arrives. Why do most people continue to procrastinate? This is why:

The vast majority of the people are in the grip of their Acquired Self, which is the virtual world in their head, an *offspring* of the collective human virtual world. That's why they stay *lost* in all of the activities of the virtual world. Most of these activities are centered around job, socialization and entertainment. Even when you have some time, say after retirement, you are likely to fill up this time with more activities of entertainment, pleasure and socialization.

Have you ever pondered where your time goes? Take an honest look at your activities. Then, figure out what activities are necessary and what are unnecessary. For example, your job is necessary, but spending time on social media on the internet is unnecessary.

Most people can free up some time for exercise if they want to. Do some exercise right now! Take a break from reading this book and go for a walk.

Chapter **13**

# Vitamins And Minerals

# For Diabetes

Vitamins and minerals have been extensively used in diabetics. Most *mainstream* physicians in the U.S. have totally ignored these vitamins and minerals. Alternative medicine on the other hand, has made *exuberant* claims about their efficacy. I reviewed the published data about these vitamins and minerals and have taken a "middle of the road" approach.

By themselves, vitamins and herbs may *not* provide adequate treatment, but they are certainly helpful as an adjunctive therapy. According to published data, the following vitamins/minerals appear to *reduce* insulin resistance. Therefore, I recommend them as an *adjunctive* therapy for my diabetic patients.

## Alpha-Lipoic Acid

Alpha-Lipoic Acid is normally produced in small quantities in the cells and helps in normal metabolism of glucose. In pharmacologic doses, it functions as a strong anti-oxidant. Cells of diabetic patients are under a tremendous amount of oxidative stress. That's why it makes perfect sense to use Alpha-Lipoic Acid as a supplement for diabetics.

Based upon a number of scientific studies, Alpha-Lipoic Acid appears to decrease insulin resistance and helps peripheral neuropathy in diabetic patients.

In a multicenter, randomized, double-blind, placebo-controlled trial (1), researchers gave three daily doses of Alpha-Lipoic Acid (600 mg dose, 1200 mg dose or 1800 mg dose) to 181 diabetic patients with peripheral neuropathy. They concluded that treatment with Alpha-Lipoic Acid for 5 weeks improved symptoms of neuropathy. They also observed that an oral dose of 600 mg once a day appears to provide the optimum benefits. Increasing the dose to 1200 mg or 1800 mg was *not* associated with *further* improvement of neuropathy.

Alpha-Lipoic Acid has *even* been given intravenously in clinical trials with significant improvement in peripheral neuropathy, and without any significant side-effects. In a study (2), researchers critically evaluated the results of Four placebo-controlled clinical trials (ALADIN I, ALADIN III, SYDNEY, NATHAN II), with a total of 2258 patients. They concluded that treatment with Alpha-Lipoic Acid (600 mg/day intravenously) over 3 weeks is safe and significantly improves peripheral neuropathy.

In my own extensive experience at the Jamila Diabetes and Endocrine Medical Center, Alpha-Lipoic Acid has been found to be effective and safe in treating peripheral neuropathy. The usual dose that I use in my patients is 600 mg per day.

# Chromium Picolinate

Chromium picolinate is required for the normal metabolism of glucose. In large doses, Chromium picolinate has been shown to improve glucose control in diabetics by decreasing insulin resistance.

Several studies have shown beneficial effects of chromium supplementation in diabetic patients. In one such study (3), researchers investigated the effect of Chromium picolinate in Chinese individuals with Type 2 diabetes. For four months, one group received Chromium picolinate 100 micrograms twice a day, the second group received Chromium picolinate 500 micrograms twice a day and the third group received a placebo. Researchers noted *significant* improvements in glucose control as evidenced by fasting blood glucose, post-meal blood glucose and Hemoglobin A1c in the diabetics receiving 500 micrograms twice per day. There were *less* improvements in the group receiving 100 micrograms twice per day. In addition, there was improvement in insulin resistance and cholesterol level.

In a study (4), researchers evaluated *twenty-five* randomized, controlled trials and concluded that Chromium supplementation, at a dose of more than 200 micrograms per day, has a *favorable* effect on glucose control in diabetic patients. In addition, Chromium picolinate appears to lower triglycerides and raise HDL cholesterol (the good cholesterol), by decreasing insulin resistance. Moreover, Chromium supplementation was found to be safe.

I have been using Chromium picolinate in my Type 2 diabetic patients at the Jamila Diabetes And Endocrine Medical Center since 2004. I have found it to be *effective* and *safe* in treating Type 2 diabetics. The usual dose that I use in my patients is <u>800</u> microgram per day.

# Vanadium

Vanadium is an essential trace element occurring in most mammalian cells. The main source of vanadium intake is food. Vanadium is well known to be beneficial for diabetics. It acts as an insulin-like agent.

In an experimental study in Type 2 diabetic mice, researchers found that oral administration of vanadium for 3 weeks decreased blood glucose level from 236 mg/dl to 143 mg/dl.

In a well-designed clinical study (6), researchers gave vanadium, as vanadyl sulfate, at a dose of 100 mg per day for 3 weeks to six Type 2 diabetics. These patients were already on treatment with diet and sulfonylurea drugs. Their diabetes was quite uncontrolled, with fasting blood glucose of 210 mg/dl and HbA1c of 9.6 . After 3 weeks of vanadium, there was a *modest* improvement in the fasting blood glucose. It came down to 181 mg/dl from 210 mg/dl. More importantly, vanadium *decreased* insulin resistance at all three levels: liver, muscles and fat.

In another study (7), researchers compared the effects of a dose of 100 mg per day of vanadium (as vanadyl sulfate) in moderately obese Type 2 diabetics versus non-diabetics. They found that vanadium decreased insulin resistance *only* in the diabetics, but *not* in the non-diabetics.

# Coenzyme Q 10 (Co Q 10)

Coenzyme Q10 is a strong antioxidant. It improves diastolic dysfunction of the heart in patients with hypertension, which is commonly present in patients with diabetes.

Can Co Q10 lower blood glucose?  In a clinical study (8), researchers asked this question. They added a dose of Co Q10 at 200 mg per day to conventional glucose-lowering drugs in 9 diabetic patients.  After a period of 12 weeks, researchers observed a statistically significant improvement in hemoglobin A1C, which dropped from a mean of 7.1% to 6.8% (a decrease of - 0.3). The authors concluded that Co Q10 improves diabetic control by improving insulin secretion without any adverse effects.

In another study (9), researchers gave a dose of  Co Q10 at 200 mg per day to 74 diabetic patients. They also observed a significant decrease in hemoglobin  A1C  (a mean of - 0.37). In addition, they also noticed a drop in systolic blood pressure (mean of - 6.1) and diastolic blood pressure (mean of - 2.9).

Co Q10 is believed to be crucial for the normal functioning of the mitochondria: the energy power houses inside the cell. Statin drugs  such as Zocor (simvastatin), Lipitor (atorvastatin), Crestor (rosuvastatin) and Pravachol (pravastatin) are commonly used in diabetic patients. These drugs dramatically lower LDL cholesterol. Unfortunately, these drugs also lower the level of Co Q10. Why? Statins inhibit the production of mevalonate, a precursor of both cholesterol and coenzyme Q10. This may be one of the reasons why many patients experience muscle aches and/or muscle weakness while on a statin drug. It is not clearly known if Co Q10 supplementation can prevent/or treat these statin-induce muscular symptoms.

## Natural Sources of CoQ10

Co Q10 is highest in red meats and organ meats, such as liver and heart. Other food sources of Co Q10 include fish (such as salmon, tuna, and mackerel), walnuts, peanuts, spinach, whole grains. soybeans and sesame seeds. However, overcooking reduces the amount of Co Q10 present in foods.

## Co Q10 Supplementation

Overall, Co Q10 supplementation appears to be beneficial for patients with Type 2 diabetes. The usual dose is 100 to 300 mg per day.

# ZINC

Zinc is an essential trace element that exists in all cells and is required by thousands of chemical reactions in the body. Zinc is involved in the synthesis, storage and secretion of insulin, as well as insulin action. Zinc is also a strong antioxidant.

Several animal studies have shown Zinc deficiency to be associated with high risk of Type 2 as well as Type 1 diabetes, but there are very few human studies. In one such study (10), researchers investigated the relationship between dietary intake of Zinc, and diabetes and coronary artery disease in 1769 rural individuals and 1806 urban individuals in India. The authors concluded that low dietary zinc was associated with an increased risk of diabetes, high blood pressure, high triglycerides, and coronary artery disease in urban subjects only.

In another study (11), "Nurses' Health Study,"  in which 82,297 women in the USA were followed for 24 years, researchers concluded that  higher Zinc intake may be associated with a slightly lower risk of Type 2 diabetes in women.

In addition to low dietary intake, Type 2 diabetics also have increased urinary loss of Zinc if their diabetes is not controlled.


## Can Zinc Supplementation Help Type 2 Diabetes?

In an animal study (12), researchers gave Zinc orally to Type 2 diabetic mice for 4 weeks. They observed a significant improvement in blood glucose level as well as a reduction in insulin resistance. In addition, Zinc treatment caused weight loss and a decrease in high blood pressure (hypertension) in these mice. In another study (13), Zinc supplementation was shown to alleviate diabetic peripheral neuropathy in diabetic rats.

How about human studies? In one study (14), authors analyzed all of the published studies in humans for the effects of Zinc supplementation on diabetes and cholesterol. Compared to a placebo, Zinc supplementation caused a mean *drop* of 18.13mg/dl in fasting blood glucose,  34.87mg/dl in 2-hour post-meal blood glucose, and a 0.54% reduction in HbA1c (Hemoglobin A1C).  In addition, Zinc supplementation caused a mean decrease of 11.19mg/dl in LDL cholesterol. Studies also showed a significant reduction in systolic and diastolic blood pressures after Zinc supplementation.

In addition, Zinc is also important to fight off infections (such as common colds, pneumonia, diarrhea), heal wounds and prevent/treat AMD (Age-related Macular Degeneration.)

## Who Is At Risk For Zinc Deficiency?

- Diabetics, due to increased urinary losses of Zinc in urine if diabetes is uncontrolled.

- Elderly, due to decreased intake as well as absorption of Zinc. In addition, the elderly are usually on a number of medications (listed below) that can interfere with Zinc absorption.

- Vegetarians, because plant foods are low in Zinc content to begin with. In addition, Phytates in grains bind Zinc and inhibit its absorption.

- Alcohol consumption, which reduces Zinc absorption from intestines and increases its excretion in the urine.

- Chronic malabsorption conditions such as Crohn's disease, ulcerative colitis, chronic diarrhea, intestinal surgery, stomach-bypass surgery. These conditions cause a decrease in the absorption of Zinc, as well as an increase in the loss of Zinc in stools and urine.

- Drugs that can lead to Zinc deficiency include:

  Thiazide diuretics: the mechanism is increased urinary losses of Zinc.

  Antibiotics such as Cipro, Levaquin, tetracyclines. The mechanism is interference with intestinal absorption. Zinc can interfere with the absorption of these antibiotics. Therefore, take these antibiotics on an empty stomach to minimize this interaction.

  Iron supplements can interfere with the absorption of Zinc in food. Therefore, take iron between meals, but not with meals.

- Any chronic illness such as chronic liver disease, chronic kidney disease, malignancy, sickle cell disease, etc.

- Children in poor countries due to malnutrition.

- Pregnant and breast-feeding women

**Symptoms Of Zinc Deficiency**

Zinc deficiency causes *non-specific* symptoms such as fatigue, loss of appetite, impaired immune function, delayed healing of wounds, diarrhea, hair loss, taste abnormalities, skin ulcers, age-related macular degeneration, delayed puberty, impotence, low testosterone and weight loss. Remember, these symptoms can occur due to many other medical conditions as well.

Zinc level in the blood is the most commonly used test to evaluate Zinc deficiency. However, blood level of Zinc does *not* necessarily reflects the tissue level. Therefore, Zinc deficiency may be present while the blood test may be within the normal range.

Zinc deficiency is basically a clinical diagnosis. Consult with your doctor in this regard.

# How Much Zinc?

The recommended daily dose of Zinc for adults is 11 mg for males and 8 mg for females.

Tolerable upper levels are 40 mg per day, both for males and females.

**Good Dietary Sources Of Zinc**

The best way to get your Zinc is through selecting foods which are not only high in Zinc, but also good for your diabetes.

Seafood: Oysters (cooked), Crab, Lobster

Meats: Beef, lamb, chicken and pork

Plants: wheat germ, pumpkin seeds, nuts, especially cashews.

Cooked oysters have the highest quantities of Zinc, followed by wheat germ (roasted), beef, pumpkin seeds and cashews.

Please note that whole-grain breads, cereals and legumes contain substances called phytates which bind zinc and inhibit its absorption. Therefore, the best sources of Zinc are animal based foods such as beef, chicken and seafood.

Caution: Breakfast cereals are fortified with Zinc, but these are not good for your diabetes.

## Zinc Supplements

If you cannot get enough Zinc through your diet for one reason or another, then consider Zinc supplements. Various forms are available such as Zinc gluconate, Zinc sulfate, and zinc acetate. Zinc lozenges and nasal sprays are available for "common colds." Avoid nasal sprays, as these can cause lack of smell sensation, which can be permanent.

The label on the bottle will provide dosing information.

## Zinc Toxicity

Too much Zinc can cause toxicity. Acute toxicity causes nausea, vomiting, diarrhea and abdominal cramping. Excess Zinc intake (more than 60 mg per day) on a chronic basis can cause copper deficiency, which can manifest as anemia and neurologic symptoms.

# MAGNESIUM

Magnesium plays an important role in the normal functioning of each and very cell in our body. In particular, it is involved in energy and carbohydrate metabolism, insulin secretion, insulin action, muscle contraction and nerve conduction. Low levels of Magnesium increases your risk of insulin resistance, Type 2 diabetes, high blood pressure, heart disease, coronary artery spasms, muscle aches, fatigue, irritability, anxiety, ADD/ADHD, dementia, lupus, menstrual cramping, systemic inflammation, osteoporosis, and kidney stones.

## Low Magnesium and Type 2 Diabetes

In a long-term, prospective study (15), researchers followed 85,060 women and 42,872 men who had no history of diabetes, cardiovascular disease, or cancer at baseline. After 18 years of follow-up in women and 12 years in men, the researchers discovered 4,085 and 1,333 cases of Type 2 diabetes, respectively. In their analysis, the researchers found a significant *inverse* association between magnesium intake and diabetes risk. In other words, the lower the magnesium intake, the higher the risk of developing diabetes.

In a well designed clinical study (16), researchers investigated the relationship between magnesium in the blood and the risk of developing diabetes in 12,128 middle-aged, non-diabetics during a 6 year follow-up. Authors concluded that low magnesium in the blood is a strong predictor of development of Type 2 diabetes, among white but not among black individuals.

## Can Magnesium Supplementation Improve Diabetes?

This was a well-designed study (17). A total of 63 Type 2 diabetics, who also had decreased magnesium levels in the blood, received either 50 ml of Magnesium Chloride solution (containing 2.5 g of Magnesium Chloride) or a placebo for 16 weeks.

The researchers found that magnesium supplementation, as compared to placebo, showed a significant decrease in fasting blood glucose levels from 185 (10.3 mmol/l) to 144 mg/dl (8.0 mmol/l). HbA1c also decreased from 10.1% to 8.0%. In addition, magnesium supplementation decreased insulin resistance in these diabetics.

### The Epidemic Of Magnesium Deficiency

We are facing an epidemic of Magnesium deficiency. Here are some of the reasons for this epidemic.

- The typical western diet is *low* in food items that contain Magnesium. According to USDA ( United States Department of Agriculture) (18), only 1 out of 3 Americans consumes the recommended amounts of Magnesium in their diet.

- Phosphates in sodas, processed meats and other foods, combine with Magnesium to produce Magnesium phosphate, which is an *insoluble* compound and cannot be absorbed.

- Stress, both physical as well as psychological, causes a *continuous* release of adrenaline, which causes constriction of blood vessels, a rise in heart rate and an increased demand on the heart muscle. The body uses Magnesium to *counteract* all of these negative effects of excess adrenalin. Consequently, less magnesium is available for the rest of the body.

- Old age is also associated with low Magnesium due to a decrease in the absorption of dietary Magnesium.

- There are a number of medical conditions and drugs that can lower your Magnesium level.

# Medical Conditions That Can Cause Magnesium Deficiency

The following medical conditions can give rise to low Magnesium level.

- Uncontrolled diabetes causes an increased loss of Magnesium in the urine.

- Chronic malabsorption diseases such as Crohn's disease, ulcerative colitis, Irritable Bowel Syndrome and Celiac sprue cause a decrease in the absorption of Magnesium.

- Stomach or intestinal bypass surgery causes a decrease in the absorption of Magnesium

- Chronic pancreatic insufficiency causes a decrease in the absorption of Magnesium

- Alcoholism causes a decrease in the absorption of Magnesium

- Acute kidney injury, called Acute Tubular Necrosis, causes an increased loss of Magnesium in the urine

## Drugs That Can Cause Magnesium Deficiency:

Diuretics, especially Lasix (Furosemide) and Hydrochlorthiazide, which are so commonly used in diabetics for their high blood pressure and weak heart. These drugs cause an excessive wasting of Magnesium in the urine.

Heartburn and anti-ulcer medications, if used for prolonged periods (more than one year): These drugs include Prilosec (omeprazole), Prevacid (lansoprazole), Nexium (esomeprazole), Protonix (pantoprazole), AcipHex (rabeprazole), Dexilant (dexlansoprazole). Magnesium in diet as well in Magnesium supplements need to be broken down by Hydrochloric acid in the stomach before it can be absorbed. The above-mentioned medicines drastically reduce the amount of Hydrochloric acid in the stomach. That's how they interfere with the absorption of Magnesium.

Steroids such as Hydrocortisone, Prednisone and Dexamethasone cause an increased loss of Magnesium in the urine.

Estrogen, in birth control pills and hormone replacement therapy, cause an increased loss of Magnesium in the urine.

Asthma medications such as epinephrine, isoproterenol and aminophylline, cause more consumption of Magnesium in the cells of the blood vessels to counteract the effects of adrenaline, which creates relative deficiency of Magnesium for the rest of the body.

Antibiotics such as Garamycin (gentamycin), Nebcin (tobramycin), carbenicillin, ticarcillin, and tetracyclines cause an increased loss of Magnesium in the urine.

Anti-fungal drugs: amphotericin B, Pentamidine, cause an increased loss of Magnesium in the urine.

Certain Anti-cancer drugs cause an increased loss of Magnesium in the urine.

It's no surprise that we are facing an epidemic of Magnesium deficiency.

## Symptoms Of Magnesium Deficiency

Common symptoms of low Magnesium level include:

- Muscle spasms and cramps
- Fibromyalgia
- Irritability
- Anxiety
- Insomnia
- Seizures
- Irregular heart beat/heart arrhythmias/Atrial fibrillation
- High blood pressure
- Chest pain to spasm of coronary arteries

- Chronic fatigue
- Migraine headaches
- Menstrual cramping
- Menopausal symptoms
- Tics
- Lack of appetite
- Nausea/vomiting
- Lack of balance
- Vertigo
- ADD/ADHD
- Dementia
- Constipation

## How To Diagnose Magnesium Deficiency

There is a blood test available for Magnesium level in the blood. However, this test diagnoses only severe cases of Magnesium deficiency, because 99% of Magnesium is inside the cells and only about 1% is present in the blood.

The best way to diagnose Magnesium deficiency is through your symptoms, your eating habits, presence of medical diseases and use of medicine, as mentioned above. If you suspect you have Magnesium deficiency, increase your consumption of foods rich in Magnesium and/or take Magnesium supplements, and see what happens to your symptoms. The good news is that in general, Magnesium supplements are safe in individuals without any kidney disease. However, toxicity can develop in patients with kidney disease. Many Magnesium supplements can also causes loose stools. More on it later in the book.

## Dietary Sources Of Magnesium

The best way to get Magnesium is through foods that are high in Magnesium. Good dietary sources of Magnesium are seeds, nuts, dark leafy green vegetables and fish. These foods are also important for your overall health, especially if you are a diabetic.

Other foods that contain some quantities of Magnesium include beans, lentils, whole grains and figs.

Seeds and Nuts:

Pumpkin and squash seeds, sesame seeds, Brazil nuts, almonds, cashews, pine nuts, pecans, walnuts.

Seeds and nuts are highly beneficial for your overall health, especially if you are a diabetic. For example, almonds are loaded with good fats (monounsaturated fatty acids), and can help to increase your HDL (good) cholesterol. Almonds are a good source of Biotin, fiber and Vitamin E. Almonds and other nuts also slow down the emptying of the stomach and consequently, slow down the rise in blood sugar after a meal. Therefore, a handful of nuts after a meal is much better for your health than traditional desserts.

Pumpkin seeds are important for your prostate health. Brazil nuts are a great source of Selenium, which is important for the normal functioning of your thyroid, immune cells and prostate gland. However, too much Selenium can cause toxicity. About 1 or 2 Brazil nuts a day provide enough selenium for your body.

Note: Raw nuts are better than roasted nuts, as roasting decreases the amount of available Magnesium.

Dark Leafy Green Vegetables
Spinach, mustard greens, Swiss chard, and kale.

Fish
Mackerel, Halibut, Pollock, tuna, and most other fish.

<u>Beans and Lentils</u>

White beans, French beans, black-eyed peas, kidney beans, chickpeas (garbanzo), soy Beans, and lentils.

<u>Whole Grains</u>

Quinoa, millet, wheat, brown rice. However, diabetics should consume whole grains in small quantities, as these foods are rich in carbohydrates and can significantly raise your blood sugars.

## Magnesium Supplements

If you cannot increase the ingestion of foods that are high in Magnesium, then the alternative is a Magnesium supplement. The daily recommended dose of Magnesium is about 400 mg. In general, Magnesium supplements are safe in individuals without any kidney disease, but toxicity can develop in patients with kidney disease. Oral supplements can sometimes cause loose stools, indicating a need to reduce dosage or change the type of Magnesium supplement.

## Types Of Magnesium Supplements:

A number of Magnesium supplements are available. These include:

- Magnesium glycinate
- Magnesium taurate
- Magnesium chloride
- Magnesium lactate
- Magnesium oxide
- Magnesium citrate
- Magnesium sulfate/ Magnesium hydroxide (Milk of Magnesia)
- Magnesium carbonate
- Magnesium threonate

Magnesium glycinate supposedly has the best absorption.

Magnesium taurate is supposed to provide a calming effect on your mind

Magnesium chloride has good absorption, but contains only about 12% of Magnesium. In comparison, Magnesium oxide contains about 60% of Magnesium.

Magnesium citrate and Milk of Magnesia are also stool-softeners.

Magnesium carbonate has antacid properties.

Magnesium threonate is a newer supplement. Supposedly, it works better at the cellular level.

You can choose what type of Magnesium supplement works for you. If you develop loose stools, change to a different preparation and/or lower the dose. In general, Magnesium glycinate does not cause diarrhea.

# VITAMIN D

In the last 20 years, there has been tremendous research in the field of vitamin D. The findings are astounding! We now know that vitamin D affects almost every organ system in the body.

### Vitamin D: A Hormone

Vitamin D is, in fact, a hormone. It is produced in the skin from 7-dehydrocholesterol (pro-vitamin D3) which is derived from cholesterol. Here is evidence that cholesterol is not all that bad, contrary to what most people think these days. The fact is that cholesterol is a precursor for most hormones in your body.

Type B Ultraviolet rays (UVB) from the sun act on pro-vitamin D3 in your skin, and convert it into pre-vitamin D3, which is then converted into vitamin D3. Medically speaking, we call it cholecalciferol. Vitamin D3 then leaves the skin and gets into the blood stream where it is carried on a special protein called a vitamin D-binding protein.

Through blood circulation, vitamin D3 reaches various organs in the body. In the liver, vitamin D3 undergoes a slight change in its chemical structure. At that point, it is called 25-hydroxy cholecalciferol or 25-(OH)-D3 (or calcifediol). It is then carried through the blood stream to the kidneys where it goes through another change in its chemical structure, under the influence of an enzyme called, 1-alpha hydroxylase. At that point, vitamin D is called 1,25- dihydroxy cholecalciferol or 1,25-(OH)$_2$-D3 (or calcitriol). This is the *active* form of vitamin D. It gets in the blood stream and goes to various parts of the body and exerts its actions.

# Vitamin D Deficiency And Diabetes

Is there a link between Vitamin D deficiency and diabetes? The answer is yes. Vitamin D deficiency is linked to the risk for developing Type 1 as well as Type 2 diabetes.

## The Relationship Between Vitamin D Deficiency And Type 1 Diabetes

Type 1 diabetes develops due to malfunctioning of the immune system. Mounting scientific evidence indicates that vitamin D plays a vital role in the normal functioning of the immune system Consequently, vitamin D deficiency can lead to malfunctioning of the immune system. Consequently, your own immune system starts to attack and kill your own insulin producing cells in the pancreas, reacting as if they are invading viruses that must be destroyed. Once you are *unable* to produce insulin, you develop Type 1 diabetes.

## Evidence For The Link Between Vitamin D Deficiency And Type 1 Diabetes

Researchers have investigated the level of vitamin D in patients with Type 1 diabetes and found it to be low in the vast majority of these patients. In a study (19) researchers from the Joslin Diabetes Center in Boston, noted that the vast majority of their Type 1 diabetic patients were low in vitamin D. The study was done in children and teenagers. In my clinical practice, I check vitamin D level in all of my Type 1 diabetic patients and find it to be low in virtually all of them.

## Evidence That Vitamin D Can Prevent Type 1 Diabetes

Scientific evidence now exists to show that proper vitamin D supplementation can prevent Type 1 diabetes. One such study comes from Finland. This study (20) began in 1966 when a total of 10,821 children born in 1966 in northern Finland were enrolled in the study. Frequency of vitamin D supplementation was recorded during the first year of life. At that time, the recommended dose of vitamin D for infants in Finland was 2000 I.U. per day. These children were then followed for 31 years for the development of Type 1 diabetes.

Researchers made the amazing discovery: Those children who received the daily recommended dose of 2000 I.U. of Vitamin D during the first year of their life, had an almost 80% reduction in the risk for the development of Type 1 diabetes compared to those children who received less vitamin D.

*This is a ground breaking study*! If some drug achieved this kind of results, it would hit the headlines and become the standard of care at once. Sadly, even many diabetes experts are not aware of this astounding study even though the study was published in 2001 in the prestigious British medical journal called *Lancet*. Investigators in the U.S. continue to spend millions of dollars in their pursuit of a "drug" to prevent Type 1 diabetes. So far, this kind of research has produced disappointing results. Amazingly, they have largely ignored the strong evidence that shows the outstanding role of vitamin D in preventing Type 1 diabetes. Vitamin D is not a drug. There is no glory or huge profits in simply telling people to take enough vitamin D.

It is interesting to note that the recommended allowance of vitamin D for infants in Finland was reduced from 2000 I.U. to 1000 I.U. per day in 1975 and then further reduced to 400 I.U. per day in 1992. (For comparison, in the U.S. it has been 200 I.U.

a day). This reduction in the daily allowance had no scientific basis except the observation that this amount of vitamin D is present in a teaspoonful of cod-liver oil, which has long been considered safe and effective in preventing rickets.

In the last decades, the incidence of Type 1 diabetes in Finland has been climbing, which is most likely related to the decrease in the daily recommended allowance of vitamin D. As of 1999, Finland has the highest reported incidence of Type 1 diabetes in the world (21). In Finland, the yearly sunshine (and therefore, vitamin D skin synthesis) is much lower compared to more southern areas. Therefore, the population in Finland is at even higher risk for vitamin D deficiency.

Not only in Finland, but in other countries as well, scientists have discovered the amazing power of vitamin D supplementation in preventing Type 1 diabetes. In one such study called EURODIAB (22), researchers found vitamin D supplementation during infancy can significantly reduce the risk for developing Type 1 diabetes. This study was carried out in *seven* centers in *different* countries across a variety of populations in Europe.

## The Relationship Between Vitamin D Deficiency And Type 2 Diabetes

Is there a relationship between vitamin D deficiency and development of Type 2 diabetes? The answer is yes. Life-style factors that are well known to cause Type 2 diabetes include obesity, old age and physical inactivity. It's interesting to note that all of these factors also cause vitamin D deficiency.

Vitamin D is important for normal glucose metabolism. It acts through several mechanisms on glucose metabolism:

1. Vitamin D directly acts on insulin producing cells in the pancreas to produce more insulin.

2. Vitamin D directly acts on the muscle and fat cells to improve insulin action by reducing insulin resistance.

3. Vitamin D reduces inflammation which is commonly present in patients with Insulin Resistance Syndrome and Type 2 diabetes.

4. Vitamin D indirectly improves insulin production and its action by improving the level of calcium inside the cells.

Now you can understand the important role vitamin D plays in keeping blood glucose normal.

## Evidence That Links Vitamin D Deficiency To Type 2 Diabetes

Is there any scientific evidence to link vitamin D deficiency to Type 2 diabetes? The answer is yes. Numerous scientific studies have found vitamin D to be low in patients with Type 2 diabetes.

In an excellent study (23) researchers analyzed a total of 21 prospective studies to explore the relationship between vitamin D deficiency and risk for developing Type 2 diabetes. There was a total of 76,220 participants and 4,996 individuals developed Type 2 diabetes. The risk of developing Type 2 diabetes was nearly 50% less in individuals with the highest levels of vitamin D as compared to the lowest levels. Each 4 ng/ml (equal to 10 nmol/L) increment in vitamin D level was associated with a 4% lower risk of developing Type 2 diabetes.

In another excellent study (24), researchers measured vitamin D, calcium, magnesium and insulin resistance in 30 patients with Type 2 diabetes, with 30 sex and age matched healthy controls. Vitamin D level was significantly low (mean level of 12.29ng/ml) among Type 2 diabetics as compared to healthy individuals (mean level of19.55 ng/ml). The levels of calcium and magnesium were also significantly low in Type 2 diabetics as compared to healthy individuals. In addition, there was a significant inverse correlation between Vitamin D status and insulin resistance. In other words, the lower the vitamin D level, the higher the insulin resistance.

# Evidence That Vitamin D Can Prevent Type 2 Diabetes

Is there evidence to show that vitamin D can prevent the development of Type 2 diabetes? The answer is yes. In a study (25), researchers from Helsinki, Finland collected health data in men and women from the ages of 40 to 74. None of these individual had Type 2 diabetes at the start of the study. They followed these individuals for 22 years to see the pattern of development of Type 2 diabetes. These researchers found that people who had higher level of vitamin D were less likely to develop Type 2 diabetes. Thus, vitamin D appears to have a protective effect against the development of Type 2 diabetes.

In another study (26), researchers found that vitamin D and calcium supplementation were able to reduce progression from pre-diabetes to diabetes. This protective effect of vitamin D was similar in magnitude to other measures which have been shown to reduce the progression from pre-diabetes to diabetes, such as a weight reducing diet, intense exercise and use of the drug Metformin.

In another study (27), researchers studied 8 individuals with pre-diabetes and vitamin D deficiency. Vitamin D3 was administered as 10,000 IU daily for 4 weeks. Their results indicate that high-dose vitamin D3 supplementation reduces insulin resistance in patients with pre-diabetes.

## Vitamin D Supplementation In Type 1 Diabetics

Vitamin D supplementation is beneficial in the treatment of Type 1 diabetes. In a study (28), 80 patients with Type 1 diabetes who had 25-hydroxyvitamin D levels less than 20 ng/ml (or 50 nmol/L) were given 4000 IU of vitamin D3. Hemoglobin A1C (HBA1C) and 25-hydroxyvitamin D levels were measured at baseline and at 12 weeks.

The researchers observed that patients were more likely to achieve lower HBA1C levels at 12 weeks if they had higher 25-hydroxyvitamin D levels at 12 weeks.

## Vitamin D supplementation in Type 2 Diabetics

Vitamin D is beneficial in the treatment of Type 2 diabetes. In a study (29), researchers recruited 92 Type 2 diabetics (34 males and 58 females). Each patient received vitamin D3 as 2000 IU daily for 18 months. Vitamin D supplementation resulted in a significant reduction in insulin resistance as well as a drop in LDL and total cholesterol.

In summary, vitamin D has the potential to prevent as well as treat Type 1 and Type 2 diabetes. It can also prevent the devastating complications of diabetes such as heart attacks and kidney failure. Unfortunately, most diabetics continue to be low in vitamin D. Many diabetics are on a long list of expensive medications, but unfortunately, all too often, vitamin D is not included. Sadly, most physicians don't pay attention to the important relationship between vitamin D and the health of a diabetic patient. Isn't it time that proper vitamin D supplementation become an integral part of diabetes management?

At the Jamila Diabetes And Endocrine Medical Center, every diabetic gets their vitamin D level checked. We find the vast majority of them to be low in Vitamin D. Proper Vitamin D supplementation to achieve an optimal level of vitamin D has become an integral part of diabetes management at our medical center.

In addition to diabetes, vitamin D has a long list of incredible health benefits such as its role in the prevention of heart disease, kidney disease, dementia, high blood pressure, cancer, and osteoporosis. A full description of these benefits is outside the scope of this book. Please refer to my book, "Power Of Vitamin D" for an in depth understanding of Vitamin D, and how you can achieve an optimal level of vitamin D without the risk of toxicity.

# How Much Vitamin D ?

From a practical perspective, you don't get enough vitamin D from sun exposure and food. In my clinical practice in Southern California, I have encountered only one young lady who had a good level of vitamin D from sun exposure alone, without any vitamin D supplement. She was a lifeguard at the beach. For the rest of us, vitamin D supplement becomes the major source of vitamin D.

## The Starting Daily Dose Of Vitamin D Supplement

The starting dose of vitamin D supplement varies from person to person. It mainly depends on how low your vitamin D level is and how much you weigh. So, please get your vitamin D level checked and then use the following table as a guide to choose the starting dose of vitamin D3.

| 25 (OH) Vitamin D level in ng/ml | Dose of Vitamin D3 |
|---|---|
| Less than 10 | 15,000 I.U. a day |
| 10 - 20 | 12,500 I.U. a day |
| 20 - 30 | 10,000 I.U. a day |
| 30 - 40 | 7,500 I.U. a day |
| 41 - 50 | 5,000 I.U. a day |

Your Vitamin D dose also depends upon your body weight. The heavier you are, the more Vitamin D you need. Why? Because Vitamin D is *fat soluble* and gets trapped in fat. Consequently, less is available for the rest of the body. For this reason, obese people require a larger dose compared to thin people.

The above recommendations are for an average adult, with a weight of about **150 Lbs**. As a guide, add 1000 I.U. for each 20 Lbs. above 150 Lbs. And subtract 1000 I.U. for each 20 lbs. below 150 Lbs.

For some reason, if you cannot get your vitamin D level checked, then here is the formula you can use to calculate the daily dose of vitamin D3. Use 1000 I.U. for every 20 lbs. of your body weight.

## Pay Attention To The Units On Your Vitamin D Supplement!

In the USA, the dose of vitamin D is available in I.U. However, in some parts of the world, vitamin D is available in microgram (mcg).

Here is the conversion factor:

40 I.U. = 1 mcg

*For example:*
400 I.U. = 10 mcg
1,000 I.U. = 25 mcg.
5,000 I.U. = 125 mcg
10,000 I.U. = 250 mcg
50,000 I.U. = 1,250 mcg or 1.25 mg

VITAMIN D2, 50,000 I.U.

When Vitamin D level is below 20, an alternative treatment is to take a high dose of vitamin D2. This is usually given as 50,000 I.U. per week for about 12 weeks. In the USA, you need a physician's prescription for this dose of vitamin D2.

Now vitamin D3 is also available in a dose of 50,000 I.U.

## The Maintenance Dose Of Vitamin D Supplement

A common problem arises from traditional medical training which teaches that once your vitamin D stores are replenished, you go back to a daily maintenance dose of 600 I.U. a day. For example, if your vitamin D is very low (let's say less than 15 ng/ml), your physician will likely place you on a high dose of vitamin D2, such as 50,000 I.U. a week for 12 weeks and afterwards, put you back on 600 I.U. a day as a maintenance dose.

Most likely, in the following months, your physician won't check to see what happens to your vitamin D level on this miniscule dose. This kind of practice is based on the medical myth hammered into physicians that once you've replenished vitamin D stores, the problem is somehow cured.

Take a closer look at this myth. Vitamin D stays in your body stores for just a few weeks. Therefore, the "so called cure" of low vitamin D will only last a few weeks and then you'll be back to your usual state of a low level of vitamin D.

For this reason, I check vitamin D level in my patients every three months. What I've discovered is eye opening! In my clinical experience, the maintenance dose of vitamin D depends on the initial starting dose. For example, if a patient requires a high initial starting dose, that patient will need a high maintenance dose. Most people continue to require a high dose of vitamin D to maintain a good level. It makes perfect sense. Why?

It's the overall lifestyle of a person that determines the level of vitamin D. If a person is very low in vitamin D to begin with, it's due to life-style, which in most cases doesn't change after a few weeks of vitamin D therapy. Therefore, it's important to continue a relatively high dose of vitamin D as a maintenance dose, especially in those individuals who are very low in vitamin D to start with.

*Most of my patients require a daily dose of 5000 -10,000 I.U. of vitamin D3 to maintain a good level of vitamin D. However, some need up to 15,000 - 20,000 I.U. a day, while others need only 2,000 - 3,000 I.U. a day.*

## What Type Of Vitamin D?  D3 or D2?

Vitamin D2, also known as ergocalciferol, is of plant origin. On the other hand, Vitamin D3, also known as cholecalciferol, is of animal origin. In the natural state, humans synthesize Vitamin D3 in their skin upon exposure to the sun. Therefore, I recommend Vitamin D3, as this is the physiological type of Vitamin D for humans.

### Vitamin D: Oral (Swallowing) Or Sublingual (Under The Tongue)

I recommend the SUBLINGUAL (under the tongue) route for absorption of your Vitamin D supplement as compared to oral ingestion (swallowing). Why? Because sublingual absorption takes Vitamin D directly into general circulation, (medically known as systemic circulation), just like when Vitamin D is naturally synthesized in the skin from exposure to the sun.

In contrast, Vitamin D from oral ingestion is absorbed into local circulation (medically known as portal circulation) from the gut, which takes it to the liver first before entering into systemic circulation. In this way, oral ingestion is not very physiological and sublingual absorption is more physiological.

This point becomes even more important in people who have problems with digestion, such as people with pancreatitis, Crohn's disease, Irritable Bowel Syndrome, gluten sensitivity, celiac disease and tropical sprue. It's also a problem for people who take medications that can interfere with intestinal absorption of Vitamin D, such as seizure medicines, cholestyramine, orlistat and also for people with stomach bypass surgery, including those with lap-band procedures.

You can get Sublingual Vitamin D3 from online retailers. One such retailer's address is: http://powerofvitamind.com/sublingual_vitamin_d.html

## Monitoring Vitamin D Level

I cannot overemphasize the need for close monitoring of your vitamin D level. An individual's response to a dose of vitamin D varies widely. As I mentioned before, because vitamin D is fat soluble, it gets trapped in fat. That means there is less vitamin D available for the rest of the body. Therefore, obese people require a larger dose of vitamin D than lean individuals. As vitamin D is fat soluble, it requires normal intestinal mechanisms to absorb fat. If a person has some problem with fat absorption, such as patients with chronic pancreatitis or pancreatic surgery or stomach surgery, then they may not absorb vitamin D adequately.

During summertime, the sun is stronger and many people spend time outdoors. Therefore, the required dose of vitamin D supplement may go down a bit. In wintertime, the dose of vitamin D may need to go up a bit. However, in a lot of individuals this seasonal variation is little as they mostly stay indoors and apply a good layer of sunscreen when they do go out. The amount of vitamin D people get from their food also fluctuates considerably. In addition, some people take their vitamin D supplement regularly, while others take it sporadically.

Therefore, I check 25 (OH) vitamin D blood level every 3 months and adjust the dose of vitamin D accordingly. My aim is to achieve and maintain a level of 25 (OH) vitamin D in the range of 50-100 ng/ml.

I also check blood calcium to make sure that a person doesn't develop vitamin D toxicity. I recommend monitoring vitamin D and blood calcium level every three months. The blood test for calcium is part of a chemistry panel, usually referred to as CHEM 12 (chemistry 12) or CMP (Comprehensive Metabolic Panel). It's a routine blood test for most people who have an ongoing health issue such as diabetes, hypertension, cholesterol disorder, arthritis, etc.

## Special Situations

### 1. STEROIDS

Because steroids lower your vitamin D, I educate my patients to notify me if another doctor places them on a steroid. When someone takes a high dose steroid in an oral form, such as Prednisone, or in an injectable form such as Solumedrol, Depomedrol or Decadron, I double the dose of vitamin D3 for the duration of steroid intake. In these patients, I check their 25 (OH) vitamin D level every 2 months and change the dose of vitamin D accordingly.

## 2. CHILDREN AND TEENAGERS

Because human milk doesn't contain any appreciable amounts of vitamin D, infants who are solely breastfed are at high risk for vitamin D deficiency. Therefore, the American Academy of Pediatrics recently raised their recommended daily dose of vitamin D to 400 I.U. in infants who are solely breastfed, beginning at the age of two months.

In most children, a daily dose of vitamin D can be calculated as follows: Use 1000 I.U. of vitamin D3 for every 20 Lbs. of body weight. In addition, it makes sense to use sensible sun exposure, especially in infants and toddlers.

The teenage years are the time when most of your bone growth takes place. Therefore, teenagers need a good dose of vitamin D and calcium. In my opinion, they should be encouraged to spend time outdoors and have sensible sun exposure. In addition, they should also take vitamin D3 according to the formula provided above.

## 3. PREGNANT AND BREASTFEEDING WOMEN

These women are at higher risk for vitamin D deficiency. Low vitamin D in the mother leads to low vitamin D in the infant. Therefore, for pregnant and breastfeeding women, I check vitamin D level at baseline and monitor it every two months. I treat their low vitamin D as described earlier in this chapter. If blood levels aren't available, then these women should take a dose of at least 5,000 I.U. of vitamin D3 a day.

## 4. MALABSORPTION SYNDROMES

Low vitamin D is extremely common among people with malabsorption syndromes such as Crohn's disease, Celiac sprue, chronic pancreatitis and intestinal, pancreatic or stomach surgeries. In these patients, early diagnosis and treatment of vitamin D deficiency is important or they end up developing another disease, secondary hyperparathyroidism. For details on secondary hyperparathyroidism, please refer to my book, "Power of Vitamin D."

In these patients, I check baseline vitamin D level. I find that it is almost always very low. I treat low vitamin D according to my strategy discussed earlier. These patients usually require a large dose of vitamin D to meet their vitamin D needs. I strongly recommend Vitamin D3 as *sublingual* preparation in these individuals.

## How Much Calcium?

Calcium absorption from the intestines is dependent on vitamin D level. The usual recommended dose of calcium of 1500 mg per day comes from the era when we did not pay any attention to vitamin D and every one was low in vitamin D.

But things are changing now. If you have a good level of vitamin D, you do not need 1500 mg of calcium every day. In fact, this amount of calcium may be too much for you. That's why sometimes, your blood calcium may become slightly elevated. In that case, you need to lower your calcium intake. Unfortunately, often your physician may tell you to lower the dose of vitamin D.

When you have a good level of vitamin D (more than 50 ng/mL or 125 nmol/L), you need only about 600-1000 mg of calcium per day.

### Sources Of Calcium

Dairy is the best source of calcium, which includes milk, yogurt and cheese. Each dairy serving has about 300 mg of calcium. Therefore, all you need is about 3 servings of dairy per day. Other good sources of calcium include bok choy, broccoli, tofu, green snap peas, okra, turnip greens, kale and eggs.

If for some reason you don't consume dairy, such as due to Lactose intolerance, then you need to take calcium supplements. People who suffer from malabsorption syndrome, also need higher doses of calcium supplements.

# VITAMIN B12

Vitamin B12 plays an important role in keeping us healthy. It is involved in the synthesis and regulation of DNA in every cell of the body. In this way, it is important in maintaining the integrity of our genome.

Vitamin B12 is particularly important for the health of the brain, nerves, red blood cells, stomach, intestines, and heart. Diabetics are *already* at risk for dementia, peripheral neuropathy, anemia, bloating of stomach (gastroparesis), decreased intestinal motility (constipation), and heart disease. Vitamin B12 deficiency makes the matters worse in diabetics.

## What Are The Symptoms Of Low Vitamin B12?

Low Vitamin B 12 can cause the following symptoms:

1. Lack of energy
2. Tingling and numbness in the feet and hands due to peripheral neuropathy
3. Memory loss
4. Dementia
5. Depression
6. Abnormal gait and lack of balance
7. Anemia
8. Burning of the tongue, poor appetite
9. Constipation alternating with diarrhea, vague abdominal pain
10. Increase in the level of Homocysteine, which is a risk factor for heart disease, stroke, Alzheimer's dementia and bone fractures in the elderly. Low folic acid, low vitamin B6 and genetics are the other contributory factors for raised Homocysteine level.

## Can Vitamin B12 help prevent, as well as treat diabetic peripheral neuropathy?

In an excellent study (1), a high dose of Vitamin B12 (2 mg), along with a high dose Folic acid (3 mg) and Vitamin B6 (35 mg), twice a day for six months was shown to be *effective* in alleviating the symptoms of pain, tingling and numbness in 82% of patients with diabetic peripheral neuropathy. What was even more impressive that there was actual *regeneration* of peripheral nerves, not just the control of the symptoms. Researchers took a skin biopsy at the beginning and then at the end of the 6 months period in 11 patients with diabetic peripheral neuropathy. They were amazed to discover that there was actual regeneration of nerve fibers in 73% of patients at the end of the 6 month period.

## Who Is At Risk For Low Vitamin B12?

Vitamin B12 deficiency is extremely common.

**1.** Anyone on the anti-diabetic drug Metformin (Glucophage). It is a side-effect from the drug.

**2.** Anyone on a strict vegetarian diet, because vegetables do not contain vitamin B12.

**3.** Anyone on stomach medicines such as Prilosec (Omeprazole), Prevacid (Lansoprazole), Protonix (Pantoprazole), Aciphex (Rabeprazole), Pepcid (Famotidine), Zantac (Ranitidine), Tagamet (Cimetidine). Why? Because, these drugs *decrease* the production of acid in the stomach. Acid in the stomach is important to *separate* vitamin B12 from food, so it can be absorbed. A decreased amount of acid in the stomach leads to *interference* with the absorption of vitamin B12.

**4.** Most elderly people have a decrease in the production of acid in the stomach. Therefore, they are at risk for vitamin B12 deficiency.

**5.** Those with *atrophic gastritis*, in which there is decrease or even absence, in the production of acid in the stomach. In addition, there is *absence* of an important substance, called intrinsic Factor (IF), which is normally synthesized by specialized cells in the stomach, called **parietal cells.** Intrinsic factor (IF) then combines with the ingested Vitamin B12, which is also called the extrinsic factor. The combination of the Intrinsic Factor and the Vitamin B12 (IF-B12) then travels through the intestines, until it reaches the terminal part of the intestine, which is known as the terminal ileum. Here this IF-B12 complex gets absorbed into circulation. In patients with *atrophic gastritis*, there are antibodies which **destroy the parietal cells.** Consequently, intrinsic factor ( IF) is absent in these patients and ingested Vitamin B12 cannot  be absorbed.

6. Anyone who has undergone stomach surgery, as there is a decrease in the production of acid and Intrinsic Factor(IF) in the stomach.

7. Those who have the following gastrointestinal disorders: small intestinal resection or bypass, gluten sensitivity (Celiac disease), Crohn's disease and Ulcerative Colitis. Why? Because vitamin B12 absorption cannot take place in anyone who has disease in their intestines, especially the terminal part of the intestine called the terminal ileum, as explained above.

8. Antibiotics can lower vitamin B12 by interfering with normal intestinal bacterial flora.

### Vitamin B12 Deficiency Often Remains Undiagnosed

Vitamin B12 deficiency often remains undiagnosed because physicians generally don't think of it as a possibility.

For example, when a diabetic patient complains of tingling in their feet, physicians do all the work-up to diagnose diabetic peripheral neuropathy. They then start you on drug treatment *without* checking your Vitamin B12 level, even if you are on Metformin. In reality, peripheral neuropathy in diabetic patients on Metformin is often due to two factors: diabetes itself and Vitamin B12 deficiency. Vegetarianism adds to your vitamin B12 deficiency.

## Vitamin B 12 Deficiency Can Be Diagnosed By A Blood Test

A blood level less than 400 pg/ml indicates Vitamin B12 deficiency. In my clinical experience, patients do much better when their Vitamin B12 level is close to 1000 pg/ml or even above 1000 pg/ml.

## What Are Natural Sources Of Vitamin B12?

Animal products are the main natural sources of Vitamin B12. On the other hand, plant-derived food is devoid of Vitamin B12.

Good dietary sources of Vitamin B12 include egg yolk, salmon, crabs, oysters, clams, sardines, liver, brain and kidney. Smaller amounts of Vitamin B12 are also found in beef, lamb, chicken, pork, milk and cheese.

## Is There Danger Of Vitamin B12 Overdose?

To my knowledge, there are no reported cases of Vitamin B12 overdose in medical literature. It is a water-soluble vitamin. Any excess amounts gets excreted in the urine.

## What Are The Different Forms Of Vitamin B12 Supplements?

Vitamin B12 supplements are available as oral pills and pills for sublingual (under the tongue) absorption.

I prefer the sublingual absorption route because the absorption of Vitamin B12 from the oral cavity (dissolving in the mouth) is excellent. It bypasses the complicated mechanism of IF-Vitamin B12 complex formation in the stomach, and the healthy terminal ileum, which are required for the *orally* administered vitamin B12.

Vitamin B12 is also available in the form of an injection. You need a prescription from a physician for a Vitamin B12 injection.

# References

1. Ziegler D[1], Ametov A, Barinov A, Dyck PJ, Gurieva I, Low PA, Munzel U, Yakhno N, Raz I, Novosadova M, Maus J, Samigullin R. Oral treatment with alpha-lipoic acid improves symptomatic diabetic polyneuropathy: the SYDNEY 2 trial. *Diabetes Care.* 2006 Nov;29(11):2365-70.

2. Ziegler D[1], Nowak H, Kempler P, Vargha P, Low PA. Treatment of symptomatic diabetic polyneuropathy with the antioxidant alpha-lipoic acid: a meta-analysis. *Diabet Med.* 2004 Feb;21(2):114-21.

3. Anderson RA[1], Cheng N, Bryden NA, Polansky MM, Cheng N, Chi J, Feng J. Elevated intakes of supplemental chromium improve glucose and insulin variables in individuals with type 2 diabetes. *Diabetes.* 1997 Nov;46(11):1786-91.

4. Suksomboon N[1], Poolsup N, Yuwanakorn A. Systematic review and meta-analysis of the efficacy and safety of chromium supplementation in diabetes.
*J Clin Pharm Ther.* 2014 Mar 17.

5. J Meyerovitch, P Rothenberg, Y Shechter, S Bonner-Weir, and C R Kahn. Vanadate normalizes hyperglycemia in two mouse models of non-insulin-dependent diabetes mellitus. *J Clin Invest.* Apr 1991; 87(4): 1286–1294.

6. Cohen N[1], Halberstam M, Shlimovich P, Chang CJ, Shamoon H, Rossetti L. Oral vanadyl sulfate improves hepatic and peripheral insulin sensitivity in patients with non-insulin-dependent diabetes mellitus. *J Clin Invest.* 1995 Jun;95(6):2501-9.

7. Halberstam M[1], Cohen N, Shlimovich P, Rossetti L, Shamoon H. Oral vanadyl sulfate improves insulin sensitivity in NIDDM but not in obese nondiabetic subjects. *Diabetes.* 1996 May;45(5):659-66.

8. Mezawa M[1], Takemoto M, Onishi S, Ishibashi R, Ishikawa T, Yamaga M, Fujimoto M, Okabe E, He P, Kobayashi K, Yokote K. The reduced form of coenzyme Q10 improves glycemic control in patients with type 2 diabetes: an open label pilot study. *Biofactors*.2012 Nov-Dec;38(6):416-21.

9. Hodgson JM[1], Watts GF, Playford DA, Burke V, Croft KD. Coenzyme Q10 improves blood pressure and glycaemic control: a controlled trial in subjects with type 2 diabetes. *Eur J Clin Nutr*. 2002 Nov;56(11):1137-42.

10. Singh RB[1], Niaz MA, Rastogi SS, Bajaj S, Gaoli Z, Shoumin Z. Current zinc intake and risk of diabetes and coronary artery disease and factors associated with insulin resistance in rural and urban populations of North India. *J Am Coll Nutr*. 1998 Dec;17(6):564-70.

11. Sun Q[1], van Dam RM, Willett WC, Hu FB. Prospective study of zinc intake and risk of type 2 diabetes in women. *Diabetes Care*. 2009 Apr;32(4):629-34

12. Adachi Y[1], Yoshida J, Kodera Y, Kiss T, Jakusch T, Enyedy EA, Yoshikawa Y, Sakurai H. Oral administration of a zinc complex improves type 2 diabetes and metabolic syndromes. *Biochem Biophys Res Commun*. 2006 Dec 8;351(1):165-70.

13. Liu F[1], Ma F, Kong G, Wu K, Deng Z, Wang H. Zinc supplementation alleviates diabetic peripheral neuropathy by inhibiting oxidative stress and upregulating metallothionein in peripheral nerves of diabetic rats. *Biol Trace Elem Res*. 2014 May;158(2):211-8.

14. Jayawardena R[1], Ranasinghe P, Galappatthy P, Malkanthi R, Constantine G, Katulanda P. Effects of zinc supplementation on diabetes mellitus: a systematic review and meta-analysis. *Diabetol Metab Syndr*. 2012 Apr 19;4(1):13. doi: 10.1186/1758-5996-4-13.

15. Lopez-Ridaura R[1], Willett WC, Rimm EB, Liu S, Stampfer MJ, Manson JE, Hu FB. Magnesium intake and risk of type 2 diabetes in men and women. *Diabetes Care*. 2004 Jan;27(1):134-40.

16. Kao WH[1], Folsom AR, Nieto FJ, Mo JP, Watson RL, Brancati FL.
Serum and dietary magnesium and the risk for type 2 diabetes mellitus: the Atherosclerosis Risk in Communities Study. *Arch Intern Med.* 1999 Oct 11;159(18):2151-9.

17. Rodríguez-Morán M[1], Guerrero-Romero F. Oral magnesium supplementation improves insulin sensitivity and metabolic control in type 2 diabetic subjects: a randomized double-blind controlled trial. *Diabetes Care.* 2003 Apr;26(4):1147-52.

18.http://www.ars.usda.gov/services/docs.htm?docid=11046

19. Svoren BM, Volkening LK, Wood JR, Laffel LM. Significant vitamin D deficiency in youth with Type 1 diabetes mellitus. *J Pediatr.*2009;154(1):132-134.

20. Hypponen E, Laara E, Reunanen A, et al. Intake of vitamin D and risk of Type 1 diabetes: a birth-cohort study. *Lancet* 2001;358:1500-1503.

21. Onkamo P, Vaananen S, Karvonen M, Tuomilchto J. Worldwide increase in incidence of Type 1 diabetes: the analysis of the data on published incidence trends. *Diabetologia* 1999;42:1395-1403.

22. The EURODIAB Substudy 2 Study Group. Vitamin D supplementation in early childhood and risk for Type 1 (insulin-dependent) diabetes mellitus. *Diabetologia* 1999;42:51-54.

23. Song Y, Wang L, Pittas AG, Del Gobbo LC, Zhang C, Manson JE, Hu FB. Blood 25-hydroxy vitamin D levels and incident type 2 diabetes: a meta-analysis of prospective studies. *Diabetes Care.* 2013 May;36(5):1422-8

24. Gandhe MB[1], Jain K[2], Gandhe SM[3.] Evaluation of 25(OH) Vitamin D3 with Reference to Magnesium Status and Insulin Resistance in T2DM. *J Clin Diagn Res.* 2013 Nov;7(11):2438-41

25. Knekt P, Laaksonen M et al. Serum vitamin D and subsequent occurrence of Type 2 diabetes. *Epidemiology* 2008;(5):666-671.

26. Pittas AG, Harris SS et al. The effects of calcium and vitamin D supplementation on blood glucose and markers of inflammation in non-diabetic adults. *Diabetes Care* 2007;(30):980-986.

27. Nazarian S[1], St Peter JV, Boston RC, Jones SA, Mariash CN. Vitamin D3 supplementation improves insulin sensitivity in subjects with impaired fasting glucose. *Transl Res.* 2011 Nov;158(5):276-81

28. Aljabri KS[1], Bokhari SA, Khan MJ. Glycemic changes after vitamin D supplementation in patients with type 1 diabetes mellitus and vitamin D deficiency. *Ann Saudi Med.* 2010 Nov-Dec;30(6):454-8

29. Al-Daghri NM[1], Alkharfy KM, Al-Othman A, El-Kholie E, Moharram O, Alokail MS, Al-Saleh Y, Sabico S, Kumar S, Chrousos GP. Vitamin D supplementation as an adjuvant therapy for patients with T2DM: an 18-month prospective interventional study. *Cardiovasc Diabetol,* 2012 Jul 18;11(1):85.

30. Jacobs AM, Cheng D. Management of diabetic small-fiber neuropathy with combination L-methylfolate, methylcobalamin, and pyridoxal 5'-phosphate. *Rev Neurol Dis.* 2011;8(1-2):39-47

# GLUPRIDE *Multi*

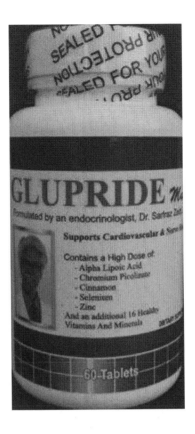

GLUPRIDE *Multi* is a unique vitamin/herbal formula, which contains **21** ingredients, including Alpha Lipoic acid, Chromium picolinate, Cinnamon, Co Q10, Vanadium and Vitamin B12. This dietary supplement is designed to promote the health for people with **Diabetes, Pre-Diabetes and Metabolic Syndrome.**

GLUPRIDE *Multi* was created by Sarfraz Zaidi, MD, a respected Endocrinologist, an expert in the field of Diabetes and Insulin Resistance Syndrome.

Call (805) 495-7143 or Visit www.DoctorZaidi.com

# VITAMIN D3

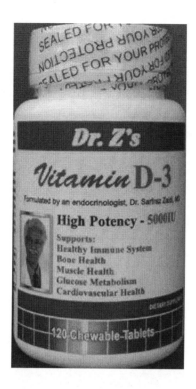

Jafer Nutritional Products,
in collaboration with Dr. Sarfraz Zaidi, MD,
now makes available a high quality
Vitamin D3 formula
As chewable tablets.

Each tablet contains **5000 IU** of Vitamin D3.

Call (805) 495-7143 or Visit www.DoctorZaidi.com

# VITAMIN B12

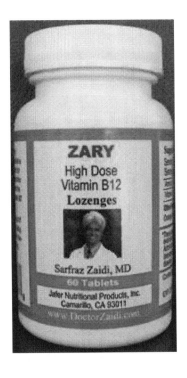

**ZARY** is a product of Jafer Nutritional Products, which is a vitamin manufacturer of the highest quality.

**ZARY** was created in collaboration with Dr. Sarfraz Zaidi, MD.

It contains Vitamin B12 in a high dose of 1000 mcg per tablet.

It is formulated as chewable tablets.

Call (805) 495-7143 or Visit www.DoctorZaidi.com

# **Magnesium** *glycinate*

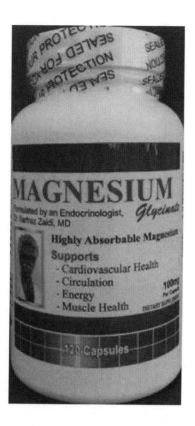

**Magnesium** *glycinate* is a product of Jafer Nutritional Products, which is a vitamin manufacturer of the highest quality.

**Magnesium** *glycinate* was created in collaboration with Dr. Sarfraz Zaidi, MD.

Each capsule contains **100 mg of Magnesium** *glycinate*

Call (805) 495-7143 or Visit www.DoctorZaidi.com

# ZINC *plus* COPPER

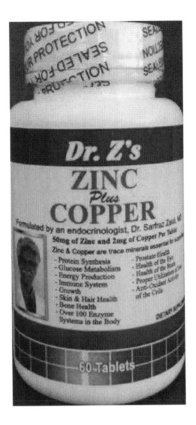

*Zinc and Copper work in concert in your cells. Excess Zinc intake (more than 60 mg per day) on a chronic basis can cause copper deficiency, which can manifest as anemia and neurologic symptoms. For this reason, it makes sense to take a Zinc supplement that also contains Copper.*

**ZINC *plus* COPPER** is a product of Jafer Nutritional Products. It was created in collaboration with Dr. Zaidi, MD.

Each tablet contains Zinc as Zinc gycinate = 50 mg
plus Copper as Copper glycinate = 2 mg

Call (805) 495-7143 or Visit www.DoctorZaidi.com

# *Dia*HERBS

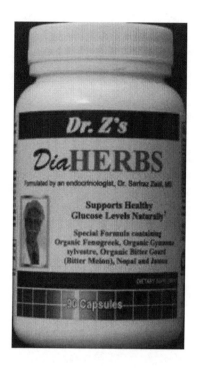

In *Dia*HERBS, Dr. Sarfraz Zaidi, MD, a leading endocrinologist has put together the most beneficial herbs in the appropriate proportions.

*Dia*HERBS contains Organic Fenugreek seed powder, Organic Gymnema *sylvestre* leaf extract, Jamun or Jamul (Eugenia *Jambolana*) powder, Organic Bitter Gourd powder, and Nopal (Opuntia *streptacantha*), leaf powder.

**Call (805) 495-7143 or Visit** <ins>www.DoctorZaidi.com</ins>

# Chapter 14

# Herbal Medicines For Diabetes

## FENUGREEK

### (Trigonella foenum graecum)

Fenugreek is used both in cooking and for the treatment of diabetes in many parts of the world, especially in India, China, Egypt and Middle Eastern countries.

A number of studies have shown that fenugreek can lower blood glucose level in diabetics. In a recently published study (1), researchers analyzed data from 10 clinical trials of Fenugreek in diabetic patients. They found that fenugreek significantly *decreased* fasting blood glucose by about 18 mg/dl (0.96 mmol/l), 2 hour post-meal glucose by about 40 mg/dl (2.19 mmol/l) and hemoglobin A1c by 0.85%, as compared with control interventions.

Clinical trials (2, 5) have also demonstrated that fenugreek treatment not only lowers glucose level, but also reduces serum triglycerides level, and total cholesterol level without lowering HDL cholesterol level in Type 2 diabetic patients.

## How Fenugreek May Work

Fenugreek seeds are high in soluble fiber, which slows down the breakdown of carbohydrates into sugar, as well as its absorption into the blood stream. Fenugreek also decreases emptying of the stomach and improves satiety. It also contains trigonelline, which acts like insulin at the level of muscle and fat cells.

In an animal study (3), researchers found that fenugreek seeds improves glucose levels in Type 1 and Type 2 diabetes by delaying carbohydrate digestion and absorption, and enhancing insulin action. In another animal study (4), fenugreek seed extract was found to act like insulin at the level of muscle and fat cells.

In an experimental study (5), fenugreek increased the excretion of fat in the feces and consequently, decreased the accumulation of fat (triglycerides) in the liver, which is a common problem in Type 2 diabetics and causes fatty liver. In this way, fenugreek may help to prevent as well as treat fatty liver.

## What Type of Fenugreek?

In one study (6), the researcher used six protocols - A, B, C, D, E and F: whole fenugreek seeds, defatted fenugreek seeds, gum isolate, degummed fenugreek seeds, cooked fenugreek seeds and cooked fenugreek leaves. The reduction in glucose level was greatest with whole seeds (42.4%), followed by gum isolate (37.5%), extracted seeds (36.9%), and cooked seeds (35.1%), in that order.

## Fenugreek Leaves May Not Be Helpful

In the same study (6), researcher found that the fenugreek leaves and degummed seeds showed little effect on lowering blood glucose.

---

## What Is The Dose Of Fenugreek?

The recommended dose of fenugreek has not yet been established. In clinical trials, the daily dose of fenugreek seeds ranged from 1 g to 100 g (median: 25 g), divided in equal doses and given two to three times a day.

From a practical point of view, I recommend using fenugreek seeds as ONE teaspoon with every meal. You can get fenugreek seeds from an Indian/Pakistani grocery store, where it is called Methi seeds. You will be surprised how cheap these seeds are.

Fenugreek/Methi seeds are hard and bitter. Therefore, they need to be cooked. Please refer to the recipes in this book to see how I use Fenugreek/Methi seeds in my cooking.

In case, you don't want to prepare your own food or don't like the taste of fenugreek seeds, you can take it in the form of a supplement.

Caution:

One has to be extra careful about low blood sugar (hypoglycemia). Long-term effects of fenugreek in humans are *not* known. Therefore, if you decide to take fenugreek, you should watch out for any unusual symptoms, as well as monitor blood glucose, hemoglobin A1c, liver and kidney functions closely.

## Any Side-Effects From Fenugreek?

The clinical studies did not report any serious side-effects from the fenugreek use. Fenugreek seeds contain fiber. Therefore, consumption of a large quantity of fenugreek seeds may cause diarrhea.

# BITTER GOURD/ MELON

## (Momordica charantia)

Bitter gourd is also called bitter melon. It is vegetable that is commonly used in many Asian countries. In India and Pakistan, it is called Karela. You can easily get it from an Indian/Pakistani grocery store.

In addition, bitter gourd has been used in traditional folk medicine in these countries for its beneficial effects on diabetes. In recent years, researchers have started to investigate bitter gourd, using the usual tools they employ to study medicines. Studies have been carried out in animals as well as humans, using juices, powders, extracts, and isolated compounds from bitter gourd.

In one animal study (7), bitter gourd supplementation reduced fasting blood glucose by 30% in rats. In addition, bitter gourd reduced the harmful effects of diabetes on the kidneys by about 30%.

In another animal study (8), bitter gourd not only lowered blood glucose, but also normalized the oxidative stress in diabetic rats.

In a recent review article (9), the authors critically evaluated the studies that were designed to investigate the effects of bitter gourd on diabetes. They concluded that some of the studies do indicate anti-diabetic effects for patients. They also concluded that bitter gourd treatment is safe for humans.

### How Bitter Gourd/Melon May Work

Bitter gourd decreases glucose absorption from the intestines, and increases uptake and utilization of glucose in the muscles and fat. It also increases insulin secretion from the pancreas.

Bitter gourd contains several substances which possess anti-diabetic properties. These include charantin, vicine, momordin and an insulin-like compound known as polypeptide-P. In an excellent study (10), Momordin was shown to up regulate the production and activation of PPARdelta, which is an important mechanism to lower blood sugar as well as serum triglycerides. Bitter gourd also contains Lectin, which reduces blood glucose concentrations by acting  at the level of muscle and fat. Lectin also suppresses appetite. In addition, bitter gourd is rich in vitamins A, B1, B2, C and Iron.

Bitter gourd is also a powerful antioxidant. This property of bitter gourd is particularly useful in diabetics, who typically have excessive oxidative stress in their tissues. Consequently, they are in great need of anti-oxidants, much more so than the general population.

### Dosage Of Bitter Gourd/Melon

The recommended dose of bitter gourd has not yet been established. Consuming large amounts of bitter gourd/melon may result in serious side-effects such as low blood sugar and its serious consequences. Therefore, I recommend using bitter gourd/melon as a vegetable as it has been used for centuries in several Asian countries. In this way, you get its beneficial effects, without getting in trouble. I have included my recipes on bitter gourd/melon in the Recipes section.

In case, you don't want to prepare your own food, you can take bitter gourd in the form of a supplement.

Caution:
One has to be extra careful about low blood sugar (hypoglycemia). Long-term effects of bitter gourd in humans are not known. Therefore, if you decide to take bitter gourd, you should watch out for any unusual symptoms, as well as monitor blood glucose, hemoglobin A1c, liver and kidney functions closely.

# GURMAR

## (Gymnema Sylvestre)

Gymnema Sylvestre is an herb, which is cultivated worldwide. In Hindi, it is known as gurmar, which means "sugar killer." In India, it has been used to treat diabetes for ages. It is also known as Periploca of the woods, Chigengteng or Australian Cowplant, in English, and Waldschlinge in German.

In an experimental study (11), Gymnema Sylvestre leaf extract given to diabetic rats reduced blood glucose by 13.5 - 60.0%.

In a human study (12), an extract from the leaves of Gymnema Sylvestre, was given to 22 Type 2 diabetic patients for 18 - 20 months as a supplement to their oral anti-diabetic drugs. There was a significant reduction in blood glucose and HbA1C (glycated hemoglobin). In many of these patients, the dose of their anti-diabetic drugs could be decreased. Five of the 22 diabetic patients were able to discontinue their anti-diabetic drugs, and were able to maintain a good control of their diabetes with Gymnema Sylvestre leaf extract alone.

In addition to lowering blood glucose, Gymnema Sylvestre is also found to decrease weight, lower serum triglycerides, leptin, glucose, apolipoprotein B (LDL cholesterol), and significantly increase HDL-cholesterol and antioxidant enzymes levels in liver tissue (13). These effects are highly desirable in Type 2 diabetics, who often are obese and have elevated triglycerides level, low HDL cholesterol, elevated Apo B ( LDL cholesterol) and high oxidative stress.

## Mechanism Of Action

The anti-diabetic effect of Gymnema Sylvestre is believed to be due to several chemical compounds known as gymnemic acids, gymnemasaponins, and gurmarin.

These compounds act at several levels to reduce blood sugar level: They reduce appetite by interfering with the effect of sweets in food on the taste buds. They also decrease the absorption of glucose from the intestines by modulating an enzyme in the stomach called GLP-1 ( Glucagon-Like Peptide-1). They also increase insulin production from the pancreas.

In an excellent study (14), researchers brilliantly showed that Gymnema Sylvestre , along with Pterocarpus marsupium and Eugenia jambolana caused an increase in GLP-1 levels. The authors proposed these herbs may have potent DPP-4 (dipeptidyl peptidase-4) inhibitory action. It is interesting to note there is a class of anti-diabetic drugs which are called DPP4-inhibitors. These drugs are very popular these days and include: Januvia, Onglyza, Tradjenta, etc.

**Dose Of Gymnema Sylvestre**

In a clinical study (15), researchers gave 500 mg of Gymnema Sylvestre per day for a period of 3 months. They observed that Gymnema Sylvestre supplementation reduced food intake, fatigue, blood glucose (fasting and post-prandial), and glycated hemoglobin (HbA1C). In addition, there was a favorable shift in lipid profiles and in other clinico-biochemical tests.

In another clinical study (16), researchers used Gymnema Sylvestre extract as 1000 mg per day for 60 days. They observed significant increases in circulating insulin levels, which were associated with significant reductions in fasting and post-meal blood glucose.

Caution:

One has to be extra careful about low blood sugar (hypoglycemia), as Gymnema Sylvestre has been shown to cause an increase in insulin level. Long-term effects of Gymnema Sylvestre in humans are *not* known. Therefore, if you decide to take Gymnema Sylvestre, you should watch out for any unusual symptoms, as well as monitor blood glucose, hemoglobin A1c, liver and kidney functions closely.

# BIJASAR
## (Pterocarpus Marsupium)

Pterocarpus Marsupium (Indian Kino Tree, Bijasar) is a tree that grows well in India. Various parts of the tree are used in Traditional Indian Folk Medicine, especially in treating diabetes.

Several experimental studies have validated the claims that Pterocarpus Marsupium can indeed lower blood glucose levels. In one such study (17), P. Marsupium decreased the fasting and post-meal blood glucose in Type 2 diabetic rats.

## Mechanism Of Action

In the above mentioned study (17), P. Marsupium significantly decreased the elevated TNF-α (Tumor Necrosis Factor) level in Type 2 diabetic rats. TNF-α contributes to insulin resistance, which is the hallmark of Type 2 diabetes. The authors proposed that P. Marsupium may exert its anti-diabetic effects through decreasing insulin resistance by reducing the TNF-α level.

As mentioned above, Pterocarpus Marsupium was also shown to cause an increase in GLP-1 levels in a study (14). The authors proposed Pterocarpus Marsupium may have potent DPP-4 (dipeptidyl peptidase-4) inhibitory action.

## What About Human Studies?

Well designed human studies are lacking at this time.

Caution:

One has to be extra careful about low blood sugar (hypoglycemia). Long-term effects of Pterocarpus Marsupium in humans are *not* known. Therefore, if you decide to take Pterocarpus Marsupium, you should watch out for any unusual symptoms, as well as monitor blood glucose, hemoglobin A1c, liver and kidney functions closely.

# JAMUN OR JAMUL
## (Eugenia Jambolana)

*Eugenia Jambolana* (Jamun) grows abundantly in India, Pakistan, Bangladesh Nepal, Burma, Sri Lanka, Indonesia and Malayasia. It has been used in traditional folk medicine from ancient times.

Jamun has been used in various alternative systems of medicine and before the discovery of insulin, was a frontline anti-diabetic medication, even in Europe. The brew, prepared by boiling Jamun seeds in boiling water. has been used in various traditional folk medicine in India (18).

There are several studies showing the beneficial effects of Jamun on diabetes. In a well designed scientific study (19), researchers gave seed extract of Eugenia Jambolana orally in diabetic rabbits. They observed a significant fall in Fasting Blood Glucose at 90 min (28.6%), 7th day (35.6%) and 15th day (59.6%). Glycosylated hemoglobin (HBA1C) was significantly decreased (50.5%) after 15 days of treatment. There was significant increase in insulin levels in the blood. In addition, there was a decrease in the total lipids level. There were no adverse effects.

In another study (20), researchers gave seed extract of Eugenia Jambolana orally in diabetic rabbits. They observed a significant improvement in serum total cholesterol, triglycerides, high-density lipoprotein cholesterol (HDL), and the total cholesterol/high-density lipoprotein cholesterol ratio.

In another animal study (21), *Eugenia Jambolana* seeds not only decreased blood glucose level, but also reduced markers of oxidative stress in rats. In a study (21), it was shown to not only reduce blood glucose, but also to protect kidneys in diabetic rats. In another study (22), it was shown to reduce oxidative stress in diabetic rats.

## How About Human Studies?

In an excellent, placebo-controlled, prospective clinical study (23), researchers investigated the effects of *Eugenia Jambolana* seeds in Type 2 diabetic patients. They had three groups: 10 patients on no anti-diabetes drugs, 10 patients taking oral hypoglycemic drugs (with history of inadequate control) and a control group of non-diabetics.

Each group was given dry powdered seeds of Eugenia Jambolana for fourteen days. On the 15th day, fasting blood and urine samples for glucose were taken. Then, there was a wash-out period of 1 week, after which blood and urine samples were drawn. Then, these patients were given *extract* of Eugenia Jambolana seeds for 14 days. On the 15th day, blood and urine samples of glucose were taken. After a wash-out period of one-week, fasting blood and urine samples for the monitoring of glucose level were again taken from these patients. These patients were then given *alcoholic extract* of the Eugenia Jambolana seeds for 14 days. On the 15th day, blood and urine samples of glucose were taken.

Out of ten patients, five received a low dose (2 grams thrice daily) and five received a high dose (4 grams thrice daily).

Six healthy subjects were kept as control: Three subjects received a low dose and three subjects received a high dose of powdered, aqueous and alcoholic extracts of seeds of Eugenia Jambolana as described above.

The results were impressive. In every patient, there was a *marked* decrease in fasting blood glucose, in both low-dose and high-dose groups, in patients on anti-diabetic drugs as well as in patents on *no* anti-diabetic drugs. Moreover, there was no decrease in the blood sugar of normal, non-diabetic individuals.

No individual experienced any side-effects except for mild headaches, which authors attributed to as psychosomatic in nature. No one experienced low blood sugar. This is the description of an ideal anti-diabetic agent: Control blood sugar when it is high, without causing low blood sugar.

The commonly used plant parts of the Jamun tree to treat diabetes are seeds, fruits and bark. Seeds seem to possess the most anti-diabetic activity, whereas leaves appear to have *no* anti-diabetic activity. In addition to diabetes, this tree is also used to treat a variety of ailments such as high blood pressure, high cholesterol, peptic ulcer, bacterial infections, etc.

## How Jamun May Work

Jamun likely acts by several mechanisms. It seems to decrease the absorption of glucose from the stomach and intestine, through acting as a DPP-4 inhibitor as was shown in an animal study (14), mentioned above. In addition, it also seems to increase insulin level and decrease oxidative stress.

## Dosage Of Jamun

Based on the above mentioned clinical study, Jamun seeds can be used as dried powder, or an extract. The dose for anti-diabetic effects appears to be 2 grams three times a day.

## Caution:

Long-term effects of jamun in humans are *not* known. Therefore, if you decide to take jamun, you should watch out for any unusual symptoms, as well as monitor blood glucose, hemoglobin A1c, liver and kidney functions closely.

# GINGER

## (Zingiber Officinale)

Ginger root has traditionally been used in many Asian countries as a spice/condiment, as well as for medicinal purposes such as diabetes, common colds, fever, muscle sprain, arthritis, motion sickness, cancer, etc. In recent years, there has been a great interest in the medical community about the health benefits of ginger. Recently, there has been a number of studies, animal as well as human, showing tremendous health benefits of ginger for diabetes, arthritis, cancer and cardiovascular health.

For example, in an excellent study (24), researchers enrolled 88 Type 2 diabetic patients. They divided them into two groups: Ginger group and Placebo group. The ginger group received ginger as 3 one-gram capsules daily to diabetic patients for 8 weeks. The placebo group received 3 one-gram dummy capsules daily for 8 weeks. At the end of 8 weeks, there was a significant decrease in fasting blood glucose, Hemoglobin A1C and insulin resistance in the group that received ginger, compared to the placebo group.

In another study (25), researchers enrolled 70 Type 2 diabetic patients and divided them into two groups. One group received a daily dose of 1600 mg ginger, while the other group received 1600 mg of placebo for 12 weeks. Compared with the placebo group, ginger significantly reduced fasting blood glucose, hemoglobin A1C, insulin resistance, triglyceride, total cholesterol, CRP (C-Reactive Protein) and PGE2 (Prostaglandin E2). CRP and PGE2 are markers for inflammation, which is extremely common in diabetic patients and indicates risk for cardiovascular events such as heart attack and stroke.

## How Ginger May Work

Ginger contains several compounds such as gingerols, shogaols, paradols and zingerone, which have been shown to possess anti-diabetic, anti-lipidemic, anti-inflammatory, anti-vomiting, and anti-carcinogenic properties. Ginger is also a strong anti-oxidant.

## Dose of Ginger

The recommended dose of ginger has not yet been established. I recommend using ginger as a spice/condiment, the way it has been used for thousands of years in several Asian countries.

In case, you don't want to prepare your own food or don't like the taste of ginger, you can take ginger in the form of a supplement.

Caution:

If you decide to take ginger, you should watch out for any unusual symptoms, as well as monitor blood glucose, hemoglobin A1c, liver and kidney functions closely.

# CINNAMON

Physicians have long been intrigued by the beneficial effects of cinnamon. In December 2003, an excellent study was published in *Diabetes Care*. In this study (26), the investigators divided a total of 60 Type 2 diabetic patients into six groups. Group 1, 2 and 3 were given cinnamon powder in a daily dose of 1 gram, 3 grams and 6 grams respectively. Group 4, 5 and 6 received placebo capsules. At the end of 40 days, there was a decrease of 18 - 29 % in fasting blood glucose in Cinnamon-treated patients, as compared with placebo groups.

In addition, Cinnamon also decreased serum triglycerides by 23 - 30 %. Patients consuming 6 grams of cinnamon powder appeared to have achieved results earlier, but by 40 days, all doses had the same efficacy.

Caution:

Long-term effects of cinnamon in humans are *not* known. Therefore, if you decide to take cinnamon, you should watch out for any unusual symptoms, as well as monitor blood glucose, hemoglobin A1c, liver and kidney functions closely.

# NOPAL

## (Opuntia Streptacantha)

Nopal (Opuntia Streptacantha) or the prickly pear cactus has been used for glucose control by Mexicans for centuries. Studies have reported improvement in glucose control and a decrease in insulin level indicating a decrease in insulin resistance.

One such excellent study (27) was carried out in three groups of patients with Type 2 diabetes. Group one (16 patients) ingested 500 grams of broiled nopal stems. Group 2 (10 patients) received only 400 ml of water as a control test. Three tests were performed on group 3 (6 patients): one with nopal, a second with water and a third with ingestion of 500 grams broiled squash. Researchers found that serum glucose and serum insulin levels decreased significantly in groups 1 and 3, whereas no similar changes were noticed in group 2. The mean reduction of glucose reached 17% of basal values at 180 minutes in group 1 and 16% in group 3; The reduction of serum insulin at 180 minutes reached 50% in group 1 and 40% in group 3. This study shows that the stems of Nopal (O. streptacantha Lem.) lowers blood glucose as well as insulin level in patients with Type 2 diabetes. The mechanism of this effect is a reduction in insulin resistance.

It appears that heating nopal is necessary to obtain the glucose-lowering effect. In one study (28), crude extracts did not cause a significant decrease of blood glucose, and the results were similar to the water control test .The intake of broiled nopal stems caused a significant decrease of blood glucose level, that reached a mean of 48 mg/dl lower than basal values at 180 minutes.

The glucose-lowering effect of nopal is seen between two to six hours after the ingestion of 500 grams of broiled nopal stems (29).

## What Dose Of Nopal?

An excellent study (30) looked at the various doses of nopal in Type 2 diabetic patients. Researchers found a direct correlation between various doses and the glucose-lowering effect of nopal. They noticed a (mean) decrease in blood glucose of 2, 10, 30 and 46 mg/dl less than basal value with 0, 100, 300 and 500 grams of nopal respectively.

Caution:

One has to be extra careful about low blood sugar (hypoglycemia). Long-term effects of nopal in humans are *not* known. Therefore, if you decide to take nopal, you should watch out for any unusual symptoms, as well as monitor blood glucose, hemoglobin A1c, liver and kidney functions closely.

# KUNTH

## (Psacalium peltatum)

Psacalium Peltatum is a medicinal plant, which is used in the treatment of diabetes in Mexico.

Scientific research confirms its anti-diabetic effects. In one such study (31), a water preparation of this plant caused a decrease in the blood glucose levels in mice.

### Mechanism of Action

It has been demonstrated that Psacalium Peltatum (AP-fraction) roots contains a carbohydrate-type compound with blood glucose-lowering property (32).

In another study (33),researchers showed that the a water preparation from Psacalium Peltatum (AP-fraction), not only lowered blood glucose in mice, but also showed antioxidant and anti-inflammatory properties. The researchers concluded that Psacalium Peltatum may be valuable in preventing insulin resistance, as well as the development and progression of diabetic complications caused by chronic inflammation.

An experimental study (34) in rabbits demonstrated that some pancreatic function or the presence of insulin is required for the glucose-lowering activity of this plant.

## What Dose of Psacalium peltatum (Kunth)

The safe, effective dose of Psacalium peltatum (Kunth) has *not* been determined for human use. Perhaps the best way is how it is used in folk medicine in Mexico, as a water preparation of its roots.

Caution:

One has to be extra careful about low blood sugar (hypoglycemia). Long-term effects of of Psacalium peltatum (Kunth), in humans are *not* known. Therefore, if you decide to take Psacalium peltatum (Kunth), you should watch out for any unusual symptoms, as well as monitor blood glucose, hemoglobin A1c, liver and kidney functions closely.

# CUCURBITA Ficifolia

Cucurbita Ficifolia Bouché (C. ficifolia) is a pumpkin-type plant, commonly cultivated in Mexico and Latin America. It is also cultivated in Asia. Its various names in English include: Siam pumpkin, Thai marrow, Thin Vermicelli pumpkin, Asian pumpkin, fig-leaf gourd, shark fin melon, black seeded melon, pie melon (in Australia and New Zealand), Malabar gourd or squash. It also has several names in local languages in Latin America and Asia.

Cucurbita Ficifolia is used in folk medicine to treat diabetes. Several experimental and clinical studies have shown that the fruit from Cucurbita Ficifolia does possess significant blood-glucose lowering effects.

One such study (34), was carried out in diabetic rats. Oral administration of the fruit extract for 30 days resulted in a significant reduction in blood glucose, glycosylated hemoglobin (HbA1C), and an increase in plasma insulin level.

In a Clinical study (35), Type 2 diabetic patients were given raw extract of Cucurbita Ficifolia or water in a single dose of 4 ml/Kg body weight, in two different sessions at least separated by 1 week. The patients had stopped their pharmacologic medication 24 hours prior to each part of the study. The oral administration of C. ficifolia was followed by a significant decrease in blood glucose levels, from a mean of 217 mg/dl to 169 mg/dl 3 hours after and to 150 mg/dl, 5 hours after the extract administration.

## Mechanism Of Action

Recently, a substance called, D-chiro-inositol was proposed as the compound responsible for lowering blood sugar (36). In addition, Cucurbita Ficifolia has been shown to possess antioxidant and anti-inflammatory properties (36).

## What Dose Of Cucurbita Ficifolia?

The safe, effective dose of Cucurbita Ficifolia has not been determined in humans. Based on the above clinical study, a dose of 4ml/kg body weight of raw extract of Cucurbita Ficifolia fruit, seems reasonable for Type 2 diabetic patients. However, it is prudent to stop anti-diabetic drugs for 24-hours before taking the raw extract of Cucurbita Ficifolia fruit, as was done in the study. One should monitor blood sugar several times a day, initially to figure out how their blood sugars respond to the raw extract of Cucurbita Ficifolia fruit. Then, one can add anti-diabetic drugs accordingly.

**Caution:**

One has to be extra careful about low blood sugar (hypoglycemia), as Cucurbita Ficifolia causes an increase in insulin level.

Long-term effects of of Cucurbita Ficifolia in humans are not known. Therefore, if you decide to take Cucurbita Ficifolia, you should watch out for any unusual symptoms, as well as monitor blood glucose, hemoglobin A1c, liver and kidney functions closely.

# GARLIC
## (Allium Sativum)

The health benefits of garlic have been recognized since ancient times. In an excellent study (37), researchers compared the results of Garlic (as 250 mg twice a day) plus Metformin therapy with Metformin-alone therapy in Type 2 diabetic patients. There were 30 patients in each group. Patients were followed for 12 weeks.

Researchers observed a significantly greater reduction in the fasting as well as the post-meal blood glucose levels in the Garlic plus Metformin group as compared to the Metformin-alone group.

In addition, the Garlic plus Metformin group had a greater reduction in total cholesterol, triglycerides, LDL (bad) cholesterol and CRP (C-reactive protein), and an increase in HDL (good) cholesterol compared to the Metformin-alone group.

Garlic contains a variety of effective compounds, such as **allicin,** which is a sulfur-containing compound. It possesses antioxidant, glucose-lowering and triglyceride lowering properties. In addition, allicin also protects against clot formation, improves blood circulation and can lower blood pressure, all of which are desirable effects in patients with Type 2 diabetes.

In an excellent experimental study (38), raw garlic was shown to significantly reduce blood glucose, insulin, triglyceride and uric acid levels, as well as insulin resistance in Type 2 diabetic rats.

In another study (39), aged-garlic extract was shown to be beneficial in men with established Coronary Artery Disease.

## How Much Garlic?

The best way is to use fresh garlic in food, as well as consume aged-garlic sometimes. If you do not or cannot consume garlic, then garlic in a dose of 250 mg twice a day seems appropriate. This dose was used in the clinical study (37) in Type 2 diabetics mentioned above.

# ONION

## (Allium Cepa)

Onions are grown and eaten all over the world. In addition, onions are known to possess tremendous health benefits such as anti-diabetic, anti-cancer, cholesterol-lowering, and blood pressure- lowering effects in folk medicines.

In recent years, mainstream medicine has shown tremendous interest in evaluating the health benefits of many plants of medicinal potential, including onions.

In a clinical study (40), Onion was given as fresh, chopped, small pieces, 100 gm to Type 2 as well as Type 1 diabetic patients. Researchers observed a significant decrease in fasting blood glucose level. Fasting blood glucose dropped by about 89 mg/dl in Type 1 diabetics, and by 40 mg/dl in Type 2 diabetics four hours after the ingestion of the onion.

## Mechanism Of Action

Onion is rich in flavonoids, such as quercetin, and sulphur compounds, such as cysteine and allyl propyl disulphide. These compounds possess anti-diabetic, antibiotic, cholesterol-lowering, anti-clot, and other various beneficial biological effects.

In one experimental study (41), a sulphur-containing compound from onion, S-methyl cysteine sulfoxide, showed a modest ability to decrease blood glucose. This effect appears to be due to increasing insulin production and/or its action. This compound was also found to possess strong anti-oxidant property.

## How Much Onion?

The best way to benefit from onions is to use them in cooking in a traditional way. Eating raw onions at 100 grams dose appear to be safe and effective, as was shown in the above mentioned study (40).

# In Summary

In summary, many herbs are used in *folk* medicine to treat diabetes all over the world. In recent years, there has been tremendous interest in *mainstream* medicine to investigate these herbs. Researchers are using modern techniques, as well as modern standards, to test these herbs. Now, there is enough scientific evidence for many of these herbs to be effective in lowering blood sugar level in laboratory animals, as described in this chapter. However, there are only a few clinical studies in diabetic patients, which are usually short-term. Clinical studies with long-term data are even more rare.

Therefore, if you decide to include herbs as a part of your diabetes treatment program, monitor your blood glucose closely, let your physician know about all of the herbs and vitamins that you take and have your blood tested regularly at about 3-month intervals, for HbA1c, liver function and kidney function. If you develop any unusual symptoms, consider stopping the herbs, and see if the symptom goes away.

In the end, I cannot over-emphasize that you should keep your physician informed of all of your vitamins and herbs.

## References:

1. Neelakantan N[1], Narayanan M, de Souza RJ, van Dam RM. Effect of fenugreek (Trigonella foenum-graecum L.) intake on glycemia: a meta-analysis of clinical trials. *Nutr J.* 2014 Jan 18;13:7

2. Bordia A[1], Verma SK, Srivastava KC. Effect of ginger (Zingiber officinale Rosc.) and fenugreek (Trigonella foenumgraecum L.) on blood lipids, blood sugar and platelet aggregation in patients with coronary artery disease. *Prostaglandins Leukot Essent Fatty Acids.* 1997 May;56(5):379-84.

3. Hannan JM[1], Ali L, Rokeya B, Khaleque J, Akhter M, Flatt PR, Abdel-Wahab YH. Soluble dietary fibre fraction of Trigonella foenum-graecum (fenugreek) seed improves glucose homeostasis in animal models of type 1 and type 2 diabetes by delaying carbohydrate digestion and absorption, and enhancing insulin action.
*Br J Nutr.* 2007 Mar;97(3):514-21

4. Maleppillil Vavachan Vijayakumar,[1] Sandeep Singh,[1] Rishi Raj Chhipa,[1] and Manoj Kumar Bhat.[1]The hypoglycaemic activity of fenugreek seed extract is mediated through the stimulation of an insulin signalling pathway. *Br J Pharmacol*. Sep 2005; 146(1): 41–48.

5. Etsuko Muraki[1] Yukie Hayashi,[2] Hiroshige Chiba,[1] Nobuyo Tsunoda,[1] and Keizo Kasono[1.] Dose-dependent effects, safety and tolerability of fenugreek in diet-induced metabolic disorders in rats. *Lipids Health Dis*. 2011; 10: 240.

6. R.D. Sharma. Effect of fenugreek seeds and leaves on blood glucose and serum insulin responses in human subjects. *Nutrition Research*. Vol.6, Issue 12, Dec 1986; 1353–1364

7. Shetty AK[1], Kumar GS, Sambaiah K, Salimath PV. Effect of bitter gourd (Momordica charantia) on glycaemic status in streptozotocin induced diabetic rats. *Plant Foods Hum Nutr*. 2005 Sep;60(3):109-12.

8. Sathishsekar D[1], Subramanian S. Beneficial effects of Momordica charantia seeds in the treatment of STZ-induced diabetes in experimental rats. *Biol Pharm Bull*. 2005 Jun;28(6):978-83.

9. Habicht SD, Ludwig C, Yang RY, Krawinkel MB[1]. Momordica charantia and Type 2 Diabetes: From in vitro to Human Studies. *Curr Diabetes Rev*. 2014 Jan;10(1):48-60.

10. Sasa M[1], Inoue I, Shinoda Y, Takahashi S, Seo M, Komoda T, Awata T, Katayama S. Activating effect of momordin, extract of bitter melon (Momordica Charantia L.), on the promoter of human PPARdelta. *J Atheroscler Thromb*. 2009;16(6):888-92.

11. Sugihara Y[1], Nojima H, Matsuda H, Murakami T, Yoshikawa M, Kimura I. Antihyperglycemic effects of gymnemic acid IV, a compound derived from Gymnema sylvestre leaves in streptozotocin-diabetic mice.*J Asian Nat Prod Res*. 2000;2(4):321-7.

12. Baskaran K[1], Kizar Ahamath B, Radha Shanmugasundaram K, Shanmugasundaram ER. Antidiabetic effect of a leaf extract

from Gymnema sylvestre in non-insulin-dependent diabetes mellitus patients. *J Ethnopharmacol.* 1990 Oct;30(3):295-300.

13. Kumar V[1], Bhandari U[2], Tripathi CD[3], Khanna G[4]. Anti-obesity effect of Gymnema sylvestre extract on high fat diet-induced obesity in Wistar rats. *Drug Res.* 2013 Dec;63(12):625-32

14. Kosaraju J[1], Dubala A, Chinni S, Khatwal RB, Satish Kumar MN, Basavan D. A molecular connection of Pterocarpus marsupium, Eugenia jambolana and Gymnema sylvestre with dipeptidyl peptidase-4 in the treatment of diabetes. *Pharm Biol.* 2014 Feb;52(2):268-71

15. Kumar SN[1], Mani UV, Mani I. An open label study on the supplementation of Gymnema sylvestre in type 2 diabetics. *J Diet Suppl.* 2010 Sep;7(3):273-82

16. Al-Romaiyan A[1], Liu B, Asare-Anane H, Maity CR, Chatterjee SK, Koley N, Biswas T, Chatterji AK, Huang GC, Amiel SA, Persaud SJ, Jones PM. A novel Gymnema sylvestre extract stimulates insulin secretion from human islets in vivo and in vitro. *Phytother Res.* 2010 Sep;24(9):1370-6

17. Halagappa K[1], Girish HN, Srinivasan BP. The study of aqueous extract of Pterocarpus marsupium Roxb. on cytokine TNF-α in type 2 diabetic rats. *Indian J Pharmacol.* 2010 Dec;42(6):392-6.

18. Baliga MS[1], Fernandes S, Thilakchand KR, D'souza P, Rao S. Scientific validation of the antidiabetic effects of Syzygium jambolanum DC (black plum), a traditional medicinal plant of India. *J Altern Complement Med.* 2013 Mar;19(3):191-7.

19. Sharma SB[1], Rajpoot R, Nasir A, Prabhu KM, Murthy PS. Ameliorative Effect of Active Principle Isolated from Seeds of Eugenia jambolana on Carbohydrate Metabolism in Experimental Diabetes. *Evid Based Complement Alternat Med.* 2011;2011:789871

20. Sharma SB[1], Tanwar RS, Nasir A, Prabhu KM. Antihyperlipidemic effect of active principle isolated from seed of

Eugenia jambolana on alloxan-induced diabetic rabbits. *J Med Food.* 2011 Apr;14(4):353-9

21.Tanwar RS[1], Sharma SB, Singh UR, Prabhu KM. Attenuation of renal dysfunction by anti-hyperglycemic compound isolated from fruit pulp of Eugenia jambolana in streptozotocin-induced diabetic rats. *Indian J Biochem Biophys.* 2010 Apr;47(2):83-9.

22. Ravi K[1], Ramachandran B, Subramanian S. Effect of Eugenia Jambolana seed kernel on antioxidant defense system in streptozotocin-induced diabetes in rats. *Life Sci.* 2004 Oct 15;75(22):2717-31

23. Waheed A, Miana G.A., Ahmad S.I. CLINICAL INVESTIGATION OF HYPOGLYCEMIC EFFECT OF EUGENIA JAMBOLANA IN TYPE-II (NIDDM) DIABETES MELLITUS. *Pakistan Journal of Pharmacology.* Vol.24, No.1, January 2007, pp.13-17

24. Mozaffari-Khosravi H[1], Talaei B[2], Jalali BA[3], Najarzadeh A[2], Mozayan MR[4.] The effect of ginger powder supplementation on insulin resistance and glycemic indices in patients with type 2 diabetes: a randomized, double-blind, placebo-controlled trial. *Complement Ther Med.* 2014 Feb;22(1):9-16.

25. Arablou T[1], Aryaeian N, Valizadeh M, Sharifi F, Hosseini A, Djalali M. The effect of ginger consumption on glycemic status, lipid profile and some inflammatory markers in patients with type 2 diabetes mellitus. *Int J Food Sci Nutr.* 2014 Feb 4

26. Khan A[1], Safdar M, Ali Khan MM, Khattak KN, Anderson RA. Cinnamon improves glucose and lipids of people with type 2 diabetes. *Diabetes Care.* 2003 Dec;26(12):3215-8.

27. Frati-Munari AC[1], Gordillo BE, Altamirano P, Ariza CR. Hypoglycemic effect of Opuntia streptacantha Lemaire in NIDDM. *Diabetes Care.* 1988 Jan;11(1):63-6.

28. Frati-Munari AC[1], Altamirano-Bustamante E, Rodríguez-Bárcenas N, Ariza-Andraca R, López-Ledesma R. [Hypoglycemic action of Opuntia streptacantha Lemaire: study using raw

extracts]. [Article in Spanish]. *Arch Invest Med (Mex)*. 1989 Oct-Dec;20(4):321-5.

29. Frati-Munari AC[1], Ríos Gil U, Ariza-Andraca CR, Islas Andrade S, López Ledesma R. [Duration of the hypoglycemic action of Opuntia streptacantha Lem].[Article in Spanish] *Arch Invest Med (Mex)*. 1989 Oct-Dec;20(4):297-300.

30. Frati-Munari AC, Del Valle-Martínez LM, Ariza-Andraca CR, Islas-Andrade S, Chávez-Negrete A. [Hypoglycemic action of different doses of nopal (Opuntia streptacantha Lemaire) in patients with type II diabetes mellitus]. [Article in Spanish] *Arch Invest Med (Mex)*. 1989 Apr-Jun;20(2):197-201.

31. Contreras-Weber C[1], Perez-Gutierrez S, Alarcon-Aguilar F, Roman-Ramos R. Anti-hyperglycemic effect of Psacalium peltatum. *Proc West Pharmacol Soc*. 2002;45:134-6.

32. Contreras C[1], Román R, Pérez C, Alarcón F, Zavala M, Pérez S. Hypoglycemic activity of a new carbohydrate isolated from the roots of Psacalium peltatum. *Chem Pharm Bull (Tokyo)*. 2005 Nov;53(11):1408-10.

33. Alarcon-Aguilar FJ[1], Fortis-Barrera A, Angeles-Mejia S, Banderas-Dorantes TR, Jasso-Villagomez EI, Almanza-Perez JC, Blancas-Flores G, Zamilpa A, Diaz-Flores M, Roman-Ramos R. Anti-inflammatory and antioxidant effects of a hypoglycemic fructan fraction from Psacalium peltatum (H.B.K.) Cass. in streptozotocin-induced diabetes mice. *J Ethnopharmacol*. 2010 Nov 11;132(2):400-7.

34. Xia T[1], Wang Q. Antihyperglycemic effect of Cucurbita ficifolia fruit extract in streptozotocin-induced diabetic rats. *Fitoterapia*. 2006 Dec;77(7-8):530-3.

35. Acosta-Patiño JL[1], Jiménez-Balderas E, Juárez-Oropeza MA, Díaz-Zagoya JC. Hypoglycemic action of Cucurbita ficifolia on Type 2 diabetic patients with moderately high blood glucose levels. *J Ethnopharmacol*. 2001 Sep;77(1):99-101.

36. Roman-Ramos R[1], Almanza-Perez JC, Fortis-Barrera A, Angeles-Mejia S, Banderas-Dorantes TR, Zamilpa-Alvarez A, Diaz-Flores M, Jasso I, Blancas-Flores G, Gomez J, Alarcon-Aguilar FJ. Antioxidant and anti-inflammatory effects of a hypoglycemic fraction from Cucurbita ficifolia Bouché in streptozotocin-induced diabetes mice. *Am J Chin Med*. 2012;40(1):97-110.

37. Rahat Kumar,[1] Simran Chhatwal,[1] Sahiba Arora,[2] Sita Sharma,[3] Jaswinder Singh,[1] Narinder Singh,[1] Vikram Bhandari,[1] Ashok Khurana. Antihyperglycemic, antihyperlipidemic, anti-inflammatory and adenosine deaminase– lowering effects of garlic in patients with type 2 diabetes mellitus with obesity. *Diabetes Metab Syndr Obes*. 2013; 6: 49–56.

38. Raju Padiya,[1] Tarak N Khatua,[1] Pankaj K Bagul,[1] Madhusudana Kuncha,[1] Sanjay K Banerjee. Garlic improves insulin sensitivity and associated metabolic syndromes in fructose fed rats. *Nutr Metab (Lond)*. 2011; 8: 53.

39. Williams MJ[1], Sutherland WH, McCormick MP, Yeoman DJ, de Jong SA. Aged garlic extract improves endothelial function in men with coronary artery disease. *Phytother Res*. 2005 Apr;19(4):314-9

40. Imad M. Taj Eldin,[1] Elhadi M. Ahmed,[2] and Abd Elwahab H.M. Preliminary Study of the Clinical Hypoglycemic Effects of ALLIUM CEPA (Red Onion) in Type 1 and Type 2 Diabetic Patients. *Environ Health Insights*. 2010; 4: 71–77.

41. Kumari K[1], Augusti KT. Antidiabetic and antioxidant effects of S-methyl cysteine sulfoxide isolated from onions (Allium cepa Linn) as compared to standard drugs in alloxan diabetic rats. *Indian J Exp Biol*. 2002 Sep;40(9):1005-9

Chapter **15**

# Prescription Medications, When Necessary

Now we come to what I see as the fifth step to manage Type 2 diabetes: prescription drugs.

## Can I Control My Diabetes Without Drugs?

You can control your Type 2 diabetes without drugs, if you have mild diabetes in its early stages, which is diagnosed with an Oral Glucose Tolerance Test, as I mentioned in Chapter on "My Approach to the Treatment of Diabetes. Unfortunately, most people have advanced diabetes by the time they are diagnosed with Type 2 diabetes. Then, you usually need anti-diabetic medications, at least initially. Think of anti-diabetic drugs as a "necessary evil."

It is true that every drug carries some potential side-effects, but uncontrolled diabetes can also lead to serious complications. Therefore, it is important to control your diabetes effectively.

Physicians should prescribe anti-diabetic medications only as an adjunct to life-style changes, which I have already described in detail. Unfortunately, many physicians simply focus on prescribing medicines, without discussing life-style changes with their diabetic patients.

Ultimately, it is between you and your physician whether you decide to go an anti-diabetic drug or not.

## Which Anti-diabetic Drug and Why?

If you decide to go on an anti-diabetic medication, you should discuss it with your physician: Why has the doctor chosen a certain drug and what are its advantages and disadvantages, including all of the possible side-effects.

In my patients, I focus on treating Insulin Resistance — the root cause of Type 2 diabetes — first and foremost. Therefore, I primarily utilize those anti-diabetic drugs which help to treat insulin resistance.

Here is a list of commonly prescribed anti-diabetic medications in the U.S.A., listed by their brand as well as generic names, followed by more detailed and specific information about their advantages, disadvantages and side-effects.

## Anti-diabetic Medications in the U.S.A

| Brand Name | Generic Name | Mechanism of Action | Class of Drugs |
|---|---|---|---|
| Glucophage Fortamet Glumetza Riomet | Metformin | Primarily treats insulin resistance at the level of the liver | Biguanides |
| Actos | Pioglitazone | Primarily treats insulin resistance at the level of muscle and fat cells | Thiazolidine diones (TZD) |
| Starlix | Nateglinide | Increases insulin production | Amino acid derivatives |
| Prandin | Repaglinide | Increases insulin | Meglitinides |

| | | production | |
|---|---|---|---|
| Byetta | Exenatide | Increases insulin production, decreases glucagon* secretion, reduces stomach emptying, and decreases appetite | Incretin mimetic agents |
| Victoza | Liraglutide | | |
| Januvia | Sitagliptin | Increases insulin production, decreases glucagon secretion | DPP-4 inhibitors |
| Onglyza | Saxagliptin | | |
| Tradjenta | Linagliptin | | |
| Nesina | Alogliptin | | |
| Amaryl | Glimepiride | Increases insulin production | Sulfonylurea agents |
| Diabeta Micronase Glynase | Glyburide | | |
| Glucotrol | Glipizide | | |
| Precose | Acarbose | Decreases glucose absorption from the intestines after a meal | Alpha-glucosidase inhibitors |
| Glyset | Miglitol | | |

| | | | |
|---|---|---|---|
| Invokana | Canagliflozin | Increases glucose excretion through kidneys | Sodium-glucose co-transporter2 (SGLT2) inhibitor |

*Glucagon is a hormone produced by the alpha cells of the pancreas. It increases blood glucose.

## Combination Drugs

| | |
|---|---|
| Actoplus met | Pioglitazone & Metformin |
| Oseni | Pioglitazone & Alogliptin |
| Duetact | Pioglitazone & Glimepiride |
| Glucovance | Metformin & Glyburide |
| Jentadueto | Linagliptin & Metformin |
| Kombiglyze | Saxagliptin & Metformin |
| Janumet | Sitagliptin & Metformin |
| Kazano | Alogliptin & Metformin |
| Prandimet | Repaglinide & Metformin |

Please note that I discuss only the main clinical points about these drugs, primarily based on my clinical experience. The description may not include every possible side-effect of the drug, for which you may want to consult your physician or surf it on the internet.

# Glucophage, Fortamet, Glumetza, Riomet (Generic: Metformin)

Metformin was released for use in the U.S. in 1994 under the brand name of Glucophage, although it had been in use in other parts of the world for many years. Now, metformin is also available under several other brand names such as Fortamet, Glumetza, and Riomet, as well as in its generic name. Riomet is unique in that it is available as a liquid.

Metformin primarily acts by reducing insulin resistance at the level of the liver. Normally, the liver is actively producing glucose during the night when you are asleep. In Type 2 diabetic patients, this phenomenon is exaggerated. Now you understand why you may wake up with high blood glucose even though you didn't eat anything overnight. Metformin reduces this excess glucose production by the liver and helps to lower your morning blood glucose.

Advantages

- Metformin by itself does not cause low blood glucose.

- Metformin modestly reduces serum triglycerides.

- Metformin also causes some weight loss.

- Metformin may reduce the risk of pancreatic cancer. It was shown in an excellent study, which I mentioned earlier. In this study (4) from University of Texas M.D. Anderson Cancer Center in Houston, researchers observed that patients with Type 2 diabetes who were treated with insulin were **5 times** more likely to develop pancreatic cancer compared to those who did not use insulin. On the other hand, patients who were on

Metformin had a **62% lower risk** for developing pancreatic cancer

Disadvantages

- Nausea, abdominal upset, and diarrhea are fairly common side effects due to metformin. If you experience any of these symptoms, either reduce the dose or even stop the drug completely, but only after checking with your physician.

- Sometimes, patients report a metallic taste in their mouth, which curbs a person's appetite. This side effect may work to your advantage by helping you lose weight.

- Deficiency of vitamin B12 can also develop. In my experience, this is a common side effect. Vitamin B12 deficiency can cause tingling and numbness in the feet and hands (peripheral neuropathy), forgetfulness (dementia), low blood count (anemia), and an increase in homocysteine levels, which is a risk factor for heart disease and stroke. Therefore, it is a good idea to check your vitamin B12 level in a blood test. If the level is low or in the low–normal range, start taking vitamin B12. Alternately, you can start taking vitamin B12 if you are on metformin, even without checking your blood level for vitamin B12. You don't need to worry about too much vitamin B12 as there are no reported cases of vitamin B12 overdose.

- A serious but rare side effect of metformin is lactic acidosis, a condition diagnosed by blood testing. This can occur if metformin is used in patients with kidney failure, liver disease, heart failure, emphysema, or shock. Lactic acidosis carries a high mortality rate. Therefore, metformin should not be used in the above mentioned conditions.

- You should withhold metformin for twenty-four hours after a procedure involving administration of a dye, such as a coronary angiogram or CT scan. The rational for this precaution is that you may develop kidney failure after these types of procedures. If metformin is continued in the presence of kidney failure, you can develop lactic acidosis.

- A blood test for kidney function (serum creatinine) should be performed twenty-four hours after the procedure. You can resume metformin if this test is normal.

# Actos
# (Generic: Pioglitazone)

Actos (pioglitazone) belongs to the class of drugs known as TZD (short for thiazolidinedione) drugs. It was released in the U.S. in 1999.

Actos (pioglitazone) treats insulin resistance at the level of muscles and fat, which are the two most important sites where insulin resistance takes place. It also modestly reduce insulin resistance in the liver, which is the third site of insulin resistance. As a result of reduction in insulin resistance, your body's own insulin becomes more efficient in lowering blood glucose.

Actos (pioglitazone) has a slow onset of action. You do not see any significant effect on blood glucose during the first two weeks of therapy. You will see its peak effect at three to four months of therapy.

Advantages

- Actos (pioglitazone) does *not* cause low blood glucose.

- Unlike older drugs such as glyburide or glipizide, Actos (pioglitazone) doesn't stress the insulin-producing cells (beta cells) of the pancreas. Therefore, you continue to have good control of diabetes for a long period of time and don't end up on insulin, which is usually what happens if you are on drugs such as glyburide or glipizide without the addition of Actos.

- In addition to controlling blood glucose, Actos (pioglitazone) has other beneficial effects. It lowers serum triglycerides and raise HDL (good) cholesterol. A good level of HDL cholesterol is the most important factor that reduces your risk for heart attack, stroke, dementia, and leg amputation.

- Narrowing of the blood vessels (also known as atherosclerosis) is very common in diabetic patients. That is why you are at a very high risk for heart attack, stroke, dementia, and leg amputation. Actos (pioglitazone) can reduce this narrowing of the blood vessels. This extraordinary effect is unique to Actos. In an excellent study (1) published in the prestigious *Journal of Clinical Endocrinology and Metabolism,* researchers observed a *reduction* in the thickness of the carotid artery wall in diabetic patients treated with pioglitazone (Actos).

- Diabetic patients have a high level of a substance called PAI-1 (plasminogen activator inhibitor-1). This abnormality places you at high risk for clot formation and an increased risk for clot-related events such as a heart attack and stroke. Actos (pioglitazone) decreases the level of PAI-1 and therefore can prevent heart attack and stroke.

- Diabetics who undergo balloon angioplasty of narrowed coronary arteries frequently develop another blockage after just a few months. This occurs due to the formation of a new layer of lining of the blood vessel wall known as neo-intima formation. In an experimental study (2), Actos (pioglitazone) was shown to reduce the neo-intima formation.

Disadvantages

- Some people can have ankle swelling and gain weight while on Actos (pioglitazone). This happens primarily due to retention of water. If you already have congestive heart failure (weak heart), Actos can be problematic, as it can worsen your heart failure. Therefore, it is *contraindicated* in patients with moderate to severe congestive heart failure. Actos (pioglitazone) can cause congestive heart failure even if you did not have it before. Therefore, while on Actos (pioglitazone), you should watch out for any signs of congestive heart failure, which includes shortness of breath, ankle swelling, and excessive weight gain without any excess in food intake.

- You may also see a mild elevation in LDL cholesterol, which may appear as an undesirable effect, but in fact, is not. The explanation for this phenomenon is as follows. LDL cholesterol has two subpopulations: Pattern B, small, dense LDL particles (which are more harmful) and Pattern A, large, fluffy particles (which are less harmful). Actos (pioglitazone) causes a shift from the small, dense particles to the large, fluffy particles. As the size of LDL cholesterol particle increases, the total quantity of LDL cholesterol rises. However, this transformed, Pattern A "fluffy" LDL cholesterol is less dangerous. Actos (pioglitazone) also increases HDL cholesterol. The ratio of HDL to LDL cholesterol essentially remains unchanged or may even improve.

- Some women may develop a decrease in bone density, which increases the risk of fracture.

- Some individuals may develop macular edema in the eyes.

- Some individuals may develop liver toxicity.


Does Actos (pioglitazone) cause an increased risk of urinary bladder cancer?

Some layman press and advertisements from trial attorneys make it sound like there is a strong association between Actos (pioglitazone) and urinary bladder cancer risk.

What is the truth? Let's look at the study that is at the root of all of this confusion.

This study (3) is from Kaiser Permanente Northern California (KPNC) pharmacy database, published in Diabetes Care in 2011. In my opinion, the study was poorly designed. First of all, it is a *retrospective* study. Every scientist knows that retrospective studies are not good scientific studies, because these studies suffer from investigator's bias. Like all retrospective studies, there were also a lot of bias-issues in this study as well. For example, significantly more people in the Pioglitazone-group were smokers, a very well-known risk factor for urinary bladder cancer. Many more Pioglitazone treated patients were also on insulin and sulfonylurea drugs than the non-Pioglitazone group. Insulin use in Type 2 diabetics as well as sulfonylurea drugs have been linked to various cancers, especially pancreatic cancer (4), a much more deadly cancer than urinary bladder cancer.

In addition, patients in the Pioglitazone treatment group had more severely uncontrolled diabetes than the non-Pioglitazone group. Diabetes itself causes an increase in your overall risk of cancer. The more severely uncontrolled diabetes you have, the higher the risk of cancer.

You can see the study design at the following link:

http://clinicaltrials.gov/ct2/show/results/NCT01637935?term=actos%2C+kaiser&rank=1

Despite all of these biases, the authors themselves concluded the following:

"In this cohort of patients with diabetes, short-term use of pioglitazone was not associated with an increased incidence of bladder cancer, but use for more than 2 years was *weakly* associated with increased risk."

Now let's put things in perspective.

Due to the controversy raised by this study, the prescribing information of Actos by its manufacturer recommends *not* to use Actos in patients with active bladder cancer.

Contrary to this study from Kaiser Permanente, several studies have observed a *reduction* in the cancer risk with the use of Actos (pioglitazone). In one such study (5), researchers found a 33% *reduction* in the risk for lung cancer in diabetic patients who were on a TZD drug.

In conclusion, every drug has its potential side-effects. We physicians prescribe a drug if its benefits outweigh the potential risks in a given patient. *Therefore, it is between you and your physician, if you want to use Actos (pioglitazone) or not.*

Update: The final results of the ongoing study about Actos and Bladder cancer risk did not show any evidence between Actos and risk for bladder caner.

# Starlix (Generic: Nateglinide)
# Prandin (Generic: Repaglinide)

Starlix (nateglinide) and Prandin (repaglinide) act by stimulating the pancreas to produce more insulin. The action of Starlix (nateglinide) and Prandin (repaglinide) lasts for four to six hours. Therefore, Starlix (nateglinide) or Prandin (repaglinide) should be taken with a meal.

Advantages

- Starlix (nateglinide) and Prandin (repaglinide) are short acting drugs taken only with meals. Therefore, the potential for low blood glucose (hypoglycemia), especially at night, is low. If you don't eat for some reason, you don't take Prandin (repaglinide) or Starlix (nateglinide). This way, you won't risk having hypoglycemia. In comparison, if a patient is on a sulfonylurea drug (which has a long duration of action), skipping a meal can lead to an episode of hypoglycemia.

- Prandin (repaglinide) is useful in patients who have kidney failure, because it is not excreted through the kidneys and, therefore, does not accumulate in the body in patients with kidney failure

Disadvantages

- These drugs do not treat insulin resistance, the underlying disease process of diabetics

- Prandin (repaglinide) and Starlix (nateglinide) are usually taken three times a day. Some patients may forget to take them properly.

- Although rare, Prandin (repaglinide) and Starlix (nateglinide) can cause low blood glucose (hypoglycemia)

# Byetta, Bydureon (Generic: Exenatide) Victoza (Generic: Liraglutide)

Byetta (exenatide) and Victoza (liraglutide) are similar drugs. They both act by mimicking a chemical in our body known as GLP-1 (glucagon-like peptide-1). GLP-1 is one of the normally occurring hormones (chemicals) in our body, known collectively as incretins.

Byetta got released in the USA in 2005. It is derived from a compound found in the saliva of the Gila monster, a large lizard native to the southwestern USA. Byetta is injected on a *daily* basis. More recently, it also became available as a *weekly* injection, under the brand name of Bydureon.

Victoza is synthesized in the laboratory using rDNA (recombinant DNA) technology. It was approved in the USA in 2010.

Byetta (exenatide) and Victoza (liraglutide) have several actions that include:

- Insulin production from the pancreas in response to a glucose load from food.

- Decrease in glucose output from the liver due to a decrease in Glucagon production. Glucagon is a hormone produced by the alpha-cells of pancreas, as opposed to beta-cells that produce insulin. Normally Glucagon causes an increase in blood sugar level by stimulating glucose release from the liver.

- Slow emptying of the stomach. Consequently, food moves slowly from the stomach to the intestines, where absorption of food into the blood takes place. Thus, there is a slow rise in blood glucose after a meal.

## Advantages

- Byetta (exenatide) and Victoza (liraglutide) are particularly helpful to control the sharp rise in glucose after meals.
- Byetta (exenatide) and Victoza (liraglutide) can help you lose weight.

## Disadvantages

- Byetta (exenatide) and Victoza (liraglutide) do not treat insulin resistance, the underlying disease process in Type 2 diabetics.
- Byetta (exenatide) and Victoza (liraglutide) have to be taken by injection, like insulin.
- Nausea and vomiting, diarrhea, feeling jittery, dizziness, headache, acid stomach, constipation, and weakness are common side effects.
- Increased risk of acute pancreatitis.

Because Byetta (exenatide) and Victoza (liraglutide) slow down stomach emptying, they may reduce the absorption of other orally administered drugs, such as antibiotics and contraceptives. Take your birth control pills or antibiotics at least one hour before Byetta or Victoza injections. These drugs can also interfere with Coumadin. Therefore, monitor your INR (International Normalized Ratio) more frequently while on these drugs.

Diabetic patients often suffer from gastroparesis, which is a condition that results from the effects of diabetes on the nerves that control the contractions of the stomach. Symptoms of gastroparesis include bloating of stomach after meals. Byetta (exenatide) and Victoza (liraglutide) can worsen gastroparesis in these patients.

Please note that Victoza, in animal studies, caused thyroid tumors and even cancer—in some rats and mice. Currently, it is not known whether Victoza causes thyroid tumors or a type of thyroid cancer called medullary thyroid cancer (MTC) in people, which may be fatal if not detected and treated early. The same precaution applies to Byetta.

# Januvia (Generic: Sitagliptin)
# Onglyza (Generic:Saxagliptin)
# Tradjenta (Generic: Linagliptin)
# Nesina (Generic: Alogliptin)

These drugs are called DPP-4 inhibitors or "gliptins." Januvia (sitagliptin) was the first drug in this class and became available in the USA in 2006. Other drugs in this class have become available since then.

These drugs act by inhibiting an enzyme, called DPP4 (Dipeptidyl peptidase-4), which results in an increase in the concentrations of two normally occurring chemicals in our body called incretins. These are GLP-1 (glucagon-like peptide-1) and GIP (glucose-dependent insulinotropic polypeptide). Consequently, there is an <u>increase in the insulin release</u> from the beta-cells of the pancreas in response to a glucose load from food.

In addition, there is a decrease in the glucose output from the liver, due to a decrease in the Glucagon level. As I mentioned above, Glucagon is a hormone produced by the alpha-cells of the pancreas, as opposed to beta-cells that produce insulin. Normally, Glucagon causes an increase in blood sugar level by stimulating glucose release from the liver. DPP-4 inhibitors cause a decrease in Glucagon, which results in a decrease in glucose output from the liver after a meal.

## Advantages

- DPP4 inhibitors are particularly helpful in controlling the sharp rise in glucose after meals

## Disadvantages

- DPP4 inhibitors do not treat insulin resistance, the underlying disease process of Type 2 diabetes.

- Common side effects include upper respiratory tract infections (common colds) and headaches.

- Increased risk for acute pancreatitis.

## Caution

- DPP-4 inhibitors can cause an increase in the blood level of digoxin. Therefore, if you take digoxin, make sure to have your blood level of digoxin checked on a regular basis. Your dose of digoxin will be adjusted accordingly by your physician.

- The dose of DPP-4 inhibitors needs to be decreased in patients with chronic kidney failure of moderate and severe degree. However Tradjenta (generic: linagliptin) is an exception that its dose does not need to be decreased in patients with chronic kidney disease.

# Amaryl (Generic: Glimepiride)
# Glucotrol (Generic: Glipizide)
# Micronase(Generic: Glyburide)
# Diabeta (Generic: Glyburide)
# Glynase (Generic: Glyburide)

These drugs are called sulfonylurea drugs. Before 1994, these were the only oral drugs available in the U.S. for the treatment of Type 2 diabetes.

These drugs stimulate the pancreas to produce more insulin. Their effect usually lasts for about twenty-four hours. In patients with kidney failure, their effect can last up to two to three days.

Advantages

These drugs start working immediately and are very effective in lowering blood glucose in the short term.

Disadvantages

- These drugs do not treat insulin resistance, the underlying disease process of diabetics.

- While on these drugs, your blood glucose can drop too low (hypoglycemia). Symptoms of low blood sugar include palpitations of the heart, excessive sweating, weakness, dizziness, a feeling of passing out, and even seizures and coma. Now remember, you may experience these symptoms if you're having a heart attack or stroke. Therefore, check your blood sugar if you have any of these symptoms. For more details, please refer to the chapter on hypoglycemia.

# Precose (Generic: Acarbose)
# Glyset (Generic: Miglitol)

Precose (acarbose) and Glyset (miglitol) act by decreasing glucose absorption from the intestine after eating a meal. These drugs are particularly useful if you tend to have high blood glucose levels after your meals.

## Advantages

- Precose (acarbose) and Glyset (miglitol), by themselves, do not cause low blood glucose levels (hypoglycemia).

- Precose (acarbose) and Glyset (miglitol) can help to control post-meal rises in blood glucose levels.

## Disadvantages

- They do not treat insulin resistance, the underlying disease process of Type 2 diabetics.

- If used alone, Precose (acarbose) as well as Glyset (miglitol) are weak drugs to control blood glucose levels.

- Patients frequently experience gastrointestinal side effects, such as flatulence, diarrhea, and abdominal pain; even liver toxicity can develop, especially with larger doses.

## Caution

Liver function tests should be done every two to three months if you are on Precose (acarbose) or Glyset (miglitol).

# Invokana
# (Generic: Canagliflozin)

Invokana is the "new kid on the block." It was released in the U.S.A. in 2013. It is a sodium-glucose co-transporter2 (SGLT2) inhibitor. It acts by excreting glucose through the kidneys. It is too early to report its long-term side-effects in the general diabetic population as opposed to the initial clinical trials.

## Disadvantages

- Invokana does not treat insulin resistance, the underlying disease process of Type 2 diabetics.

- Invokana may cause excessive urination, dehydration, low blood pressure, increase in Potassium level in the blood (which can be life-threatening), kidney dysfunction, increase in LDL cholesterol, urinary tract infections, and genital fungal infections.

## References

1. Koshiyama H, Shimono D, et al. Inhibitory effect of pioglitazone on carotid arterial wall thickness in type 2 diabetes. *J Clin Endocrinol Metab* 2001; 86(7):3452–6.

2. Yoshimoto T, Naruse M, et al. Vasculo-protective effects of insulin sensitizing
agent pioglitazone in neointimal thickening and hypertensive vascular hypertrophy. *Atherosclerosis* 1999; 145(2):333–40.

3. Lewis JD[1], Ferrara A, Peng T, Hedderson M, Bilker WB, Quesenberry CP Jr, Vaughn DJ, Nessel L, Selby J, Strom BL. Risk of bladder cancer among diabetic patients treated with

pioglitazone: interim report of a longitudinal cohort study. *Diabetes Care.* 2011 Apr;34(4):916-22.

4. Li D, Yeung SC, Hassan MM, Konopleva M, Abbruzzese JL. Antidiabetic therapies affect risk of pancreatic cancer. *Gastroenterology.* 2009 Aug;137(2):482-8

5. Govindarajan R[1], Ratnasinghe L, Simmons DL, Siegel ER, Midathada MV, Kim L, Kim PJ, Owens RJ, Lang NP. Thiazolidinediones and the risk of lung, prostate, and colon cancer in patients with diabetes. *J Clin Oncol.* 2007 Apr 20;25(12):1476-81.

Chapter **16**

# Monitoring Diabetes, High Blood Pressure And Cholesterol

Type 2 diabetes, along with high blood pressure and cholesterol disorder, are manifestations of Insulin Resistance Syndrome. These are chronic diseases, which can often lead to complications if left untreated and unmonitored. Therefore, it is important for you to monitor your diabetes, blood pressure and cholesterol disorder.

## 1. Monitoring Diabetes

In order to monitor your diabetes, you need to check your blood glucose and Hemoglobin A1c (HbA1c). In addition, you need to get tested for the effects of diabetes on your kidneys, and eyes. Also, you need to be checked for the effects of diabetes on your feet. You also need to learn about low blood sugar and how to treat it.

### What Should My Blood Glucose Values Be?

I tell my patients to aim for the following values for their blood glucose.

- Pre-meal blood glucose should be 70-120 mg/dl, preferably less than 100 mg/dl.

- Two-hour post meal blood glucose should be less than 140 mg/dl.

## How Often Should I Test My Blood Glucose?

As a Type 2 diabetic, you should test your blood glucose about <u>two</u> hours after each meal. For many patients, this does become cumbersome. Pricking your fingers several times a day is no fun. I tell my patients to rotate the timing of testing each day. For example, one day check it two hours after breakfast, next day two hours after lunch and the third day, do it two hours after dinner.

The two hour post-meal blood glucose value is particularly important for the following reasons:

- The two hour post meal blood glucose has been shown to be closely linked to the risk for heart attack in several excellent medical studies.

- It shows the impact of your food on your blood glucose. The two hour post-meal blood glucose value should be less than 140 mg/dl. A value more than 140 mg/dl indicates that you either ate too much or you ate the wrong food or a combination of these two factors. You should write down what you eat. Soon you will know what to eat and what to avoid. Share this diary with your doctor on each visit.

- Check your blood glucose whenever you are weak, dizzy or confused.

- Record all of these blood glucose values, along with your meal and any symptoms in a log.

- DO NOT forget to bring your log to your appointment with your physician. New glucose meters have the ability to store blood glucose values in memory.

## What is Hemoglobin A1c (HbA1c)? What number should it be?

Hemoglobin A1c (HbA1c) is a blood test that measures overall blood glucose values around the clock for the preceding 3 months.

I aim for HbA1c to be less than 6.0% in the majority of my Type 2 diabetic patients. I do it by using my specific 5-step approach: stress management, diet, exercise, vitamins/herbs and medications that treat insulin resistance. In this way, there is no/minimal risk of low blood sugar (hypoglycemia.) In my experience, patients with a HbA1c less than 6.0% rarely suffer from the complications of diabetes.

Caution:

If you were to simply focus on reducing HbA1c to below 6.0% by using any medications including insulin, then you are at *high* risk of hypoglycemia. It may actually be *detrimental* to your health.

More on "Low Blood Sugar" in the next chapter.

## Screening for Early Diabetic Kidney Disease (Nephropathy)

At the early stages of diabetic kidney disease, albumin, a special protein, starts to leak into the urine due to damage to the wall of the nephron, the basic unit of the kidneys. Clinically, this albumin leakage can be detected by measuring albumin excretion in the urine.

A urinary albumin excretion of more than 20 mg., but less than 300 mg. per 24 hours period is known as microalbuminuria. Your blood test for creatinine are usually normal at this stage.

Patients do not have any symptoms of diabetic kidney disease at this stage, which usually lasts for several years.

Please note that routine urine testing does not detect this small amount of albumin excretion.

Three special methods of screening for microalbumin excretion are available:

1. Measurement of albumin-to-creatinine ratio in a random spot collection.
2. Timed (4 hours or overnight) urine collection.
3. 24 hours urine collection. (the best test)

Diabetic kidney disease at this stage can be halted and even reversed in a majority of diabetic patients.

Diabetic patients with microalbuminuria should be treated with an ACE-inhibitor or an Angiotensin Receptor Blocking drug (provided there are no contraindications) even if their blood pressure is not elevated.

*See Chapter 22: Kidney Disease in Diabetics on page 247 for more details.*

### Evaluation for Diabetic Eye Disease (Retinopathy)

A complete eye examination should be done by an ophthalmologist or an optometrist on a yearly basis, starting at the time of diagnosis for Type 2 diabetics. For Type 1 diabetics, this monitoring should start at 5 years after the diagnosis.

*For details, please refer to Chapter 26: Eye disease in Diabetics on page 275.*

**A foot examination** should be done, for neuropathy (nerve disease), pulses, ulcers, fissures, calluses and deformities at least once a year. In addition to your regular physician, you should also see a podiatrist, at least once a year for a detailed foot examination.

# 2. Blood Pressure Control

Most Type 2 diabetic patients also suffer from high blood pressure, which is another manifestation of underlying insulin resistance.

I target blood pressure in my Type 2 diabetic patients to be less than 130/80 mm Hg. I do it by using my specific approach: stress management, diet, exercise, vitamins/herbs and medications.

I find stress management and weight reduction to be the most significant steps in achieving the target blood pressure levels in my Type 2 diabetic patients.

At the Jamila Diabetes and Endocrine Medical Center, I have been able to lower blood pressure to less than 130/80 in a majority of my patients. A number of these patients have a systolic blood pressure of less than 120 mm Hg. The risk for complications has been markedly reduced in these patients.

# 3. Cholesterol Control

Most Type 2 diabetics also suffer from cholesterol disorder. Typically, their HDL (good) cholesterol is low, triglycerides are high and LDL (bad) cholesterol pattern is B, all of which are the manifestations of the underlying insulin resistance.

In my Type 2 diabetic patients, I aim for the HDL, triglycerides and LDL levels to be as follows:

- HDL cholesterol to be greater than 50 mg/dl. HDL2 to be greater than 15 mg/dl
- Triglycerides level to be less than 100 mg/dl.
- LDL cholesterol to be less than 100 mg/dl, and its pattern to be Type A, instead of B.

I am glad to report that most of my diabetic patients have been able to achieve these target levels for cholesterol at the Jamila Diabetes and Endocrine Medical Center. I achieve these results by using my specific 5-step approach: stress management, diet, exercise, vitamins/herbs and medications.

Chapter **17**

# What is Low Blood Glucose (Hypoglycemia), and How To Treat It

Educate yourself as well as your family members about low blood glucose. If your blood glucose goes below 70 mg/dl, you have low blood glucose (technically called hypoglycemia).

The lower the blood glucose, the more severe your hypoglycemia. Most people have minimal symptoms at blood glucose levels between 70 – 60, moderate symptoms at levels between 60 - 40 and will pass out if their blood glucose is below 40 mg/dl.

## Symptoms of Hypoglycemia

The usual initial symptoms of mild to moderate hypoglycemia are:

- Heart pounding
- Cold sweats
- Dizziness
- Weakness
- Abdominal discomfort

Symptoms of more severe hypoglycemia include:

- Headache

- Foggy thinking
- Blurred vision
- Disorientation
- Feeling of passing out
- Seizure
- Coma

The drugs that can cause Hypoglycemia:

- Insulin

- Sulfonylurea drugs: These include Glucotrol (glipizide), Micronase, Diabeta, Glynase (glyburide), Amaryl (glimeparide).

- Starlix (nateglinide ), Prandine (repaglinide )

- Precose

Out of these drugs, insulin is the most potent to give rise to hypoglycemia. In order of potency, sulfonylurea drugs come next, then Starlix and Prandin, and lastly Precose.

The drugs that are unlikely to cause hypoglycemia:

The following drugs are *not* supposed to cause hypoglycemia by themselves, but in combination with the above mentioned drugs, hypoglycemia can occur.

- Glucophage, Fortamet (generic: metformin)
- Actos (generic: pioglitazone)
- Januvia (generic: sitagliptin),
- Onglyza (generic: saxagliptin),
- Tradjenta (generic: linagliptin),
- Nesina (generic: alogliptin)
- Byetta, Bydureon (generic: exenatide)
- Victoza (generic: liraglutide)
- Invokana (generic: canagliflozin)

You need to aware that the above mentioned symptoms are not specific to hypoglycemia alone. These symptoms may be due to other medical conditions as well. For example, cold sweats, pounding of the heart and a feeling of passing out are also symptoms of a heart attack. A diabetic is at high risk for a heart attack.

Foggy thinking, disorientation, headache and blurred vision may be due to a stroke or a migraine headache. Being a diabetic places you at high risk for stroke.

These symptoms may also be due to a very high blood glucose level.

## How to Treat Hypoglycemia

If you have symptoms of hypoglycemia, but do **not** have a feeling of passing out, then check your blood glucose. If it is above 70 mg/dl, you do not have hypoglycemia. Your symptoms may be due to other reasons, such as a heart attack or a stroke. Call 911, if you reside in the U.S. or go to the nearby hospital.

If you cannot check your blood glucose, and are on one of the drugs that can cause hypoglycemia, then presume you have hypoglycemia and ingest glucose in any form.(whatever is available, such as fruit juice, regular sugar, candy, glucose tablets)

If you have blurry vision, disorientation, a feeling of passing out, but are conscious, then presume that you have hypoglycemia and drink some glucose in any form.

Note: hypoglycemia due to Precose does not respond to regular sugar, but to glucose tablets.

Check your blood glucose in about 15 minutes. Usually by that time, you should be feeling better and your blood glucose should be above 70 mg/dl. Then you should also eat a snack or a meal (if it's meal time) and skip your diabetes medicine for that meal. Also call your doctor for further advice.

Hypoglycemia due to Sulfonylurea drugs and long acting insulin can recur within 24 hours. In patients with kidney failure, this dangerous period may last up to 72 hours as these drugs hang around for a much longer period.

Therefore, you should be monitored in a hospital. Alternatively, if you feel comfortable at home, continue to check your blood glucose frequently and stay in touch with your doctor. Someone must be with you the entire time you are at home. You should not drive or engage in any hazardous activity during this period.

The effects of Short acting insulin, Starlix, Prandin and Precose last for about 4-6 hours. Therefore you are usually out of the woods after about 4-6 hours.

If you become unconscious, your spouse, friend or companion should give you a Glucagon shot and call 911. You should be taken to the nearby hospital and properly evaluated.

Every patient on insulin should have a **Glucagon** kit nearby in order to treat hypoglycemia. A family member, friend or teacher should know about this Glucagon kit and should give this injection to the patient in case he/she becomes unconscious. Glucagon acts rapidly and can save a patient's life.

**Other Useful hints:**

Type 1 diabetics are at higher risk for hypoglycemia than Type 2 diabetics.

Patients with kidney failure who are on insulin or oral hypoglycemic diabetic drugs are at high risk for hypoglycemia as compared to those without kidney failure.

Some diabetic patients, especially Type 1 diabetics of long duration, can develop a situation where they become hypoglycemic without any symptoms. This is known as **hypoglycemia unawareness** and it can be life-threatening. If you have this condition, you should be treated by an experienced endocrinologist.

**Nocturnal hypoglycemia** (hypoglycemia at night) often develops because of short acting insulin taken at bed time. This can be avoided by not taking any short acting insulin at bedtime. A protein snack at bedtime can also help to prevent nocturnal hypoglycemia.

Every diabetic patient, especially Type 1 diabetics, should wear a medic alert bracelet.

*Section 3*

# Prevent/Treat/Reverse Complications of Diabetes

Chapter **18**

# How to Prevent/Treat/Reverse Complications of Diabetes

Type 2 Diabetes is a disease of complications if it is not treated properly. It's important to understand the possible complications that can arise from your disease (or that may have already arisen) and to understand the further treatment tools available to prevent, stop, or even reverse these complications..

Diabetes can affect almost every part of your body. As a diabetic, you're at a high risk for a number of complications, regardless of whether you require insulin or not. Don't be lulled into thinking that Type 2 diabetes — what many consider the "good kind" because you are not on insulin shots — leaves you at any less risk for complications. A major part of taking charge of your diabetes is to understand your risks and learn how you can prevent, manage or even reverse these complications.

The list of frequent diabetes complications includes:

- Heart disease
- Stroke
- Eye disease, which can lead to blindness
- Poor circulation, which can lead to amputation of feet/legs
- Kidney failure, which can lead to "dialysis"
- Peripheral neuropathy (Define)
- Autonomic Neuropathy (gastroparesis, diarrhea, constipation, dizziness)
- Impotence

- Fatty liver, which may lead to cirrhosis
- Increased susceptibility to infections

These deadly complications develop insidiously over a long period of time. That is why patients often don't fully comprehend the devastating effects of diabetes until it's too late. The good news — as I've stated earlier — is that my treatment approach can help *prevent* these horrendous complications.

You can also *stop* and even *reverse* the downhill course of some of these complications after they have developed. Again, the key is to understand how these complications develop and how your treatment for diabetes should include measures to stave off these complications. What follows in the next several chapters is information about each of the major complications of diabetes.

## A Message for Smokers

Diabetics who smoke have a markedly increased risk for developing complications of diabetes. So next time you light up, remember that the smoke is *fueling* the fire of complications. Read this section, and then take a moment to meditate about the path you are on. Maybe if you truly comprehend what lies ahead on this road, you can find the strength to commit to quit smoking.

Chapter **19**

# Heart Disease in Diabetics

Coronary heart disease develops due to narrowing of the blood vessels, a process known as atherosclerosis. Atherosclerosis develops slowly over a number of years. Then one day, a clot forms at the site of the narrowed blood vessel and acutely shuts down the blood flow to a portion of the heart muscle, causing an acute heart attack or technically speaking, angina (a minor episode without any damage to the heart muscle) or acute myocardial infarction (a prolonged episode with damage to the heart muscle).

The root cause for coronary heart disease in a majority of diabetics is Insulin Resistance Syndrome (IRS). Heart disease and heart attacks are preventable, but only with proper evaluation and treatment of IRS. If you have the risk factors for IRS—abdominal obesity, high blood pressure, low HDL cholesterol, high triglycerides, Pattern B LDL cholesterol, or elevated CRP (C-reactive protein), you and your physician need to target IRS and treat it.

**How Insulin Resistance Puts You At A High Risk For Heart Attack**

1. The Effects of High Levels of Insulin

A person with Insulin Resistance Syndrome has a higher than normal level of insulin in the bloodstream, which in turn stimulates the growth of smooth muscle cells in the walls of the coronary arteries. This causes thickening and stiffness of the arterial walls, which contributes to narrowing of the coronary blood vessels: atherosclerosis.

## 2. High Blood Pressure

High blood pressure, a component of IRS, is present in most Type 2 diabetics, and is known to cause narrowing of the arterial blood vessels, including arteries of the heart. Blood pressure higher than 120/80 mm Hg increases your risk for a heart attack. Blood pressure above 130/85 mm Hg is called hypertension. A healthy blood pressure is less than 120/80 mm Hg in most individuals, as long as you don't have dizziness. However, in the elderly, aggressive lowering of blood pressure is not desirable, as long as blood pressure is less than 140/90.

High insulin levels, due to insulin resistance, causes high blood pressure by the following mechanisms:

• It causes thickening of arterial walls, which then become stiff. Increased resistance to blood flow through the stiff blood vessels leads to an increase in blood pressure.

• It causes retention of sodium and water from the kidneys, which then leads to high blood pressure.

• It stimulates the sympathetic nervous system, which causes constriction of blood vessels, which then leads to high blood pressure.

## 3. High Triglycerides and Low HDL Cholesterol

A high level of triglycerides and a low level of HDL (good) cholesterol, both of which are components of IRS, are present in most Type 2 diabetics.

In healthy individuals, one of the functions of insulin is to suppress the breakdown of fat from the fat cells into the blood stream. This action of insulin is hampered in individuals with insulin resistance. As a result there is an exaggerated breakdown of fat from the fat cells. The product of this fat breakdown is called free fatty acids. Thus, in diabetics with insulin resistance, there is a high level of free fatty acids in the blood. The liver takes up these free fatty acids and converts them into VLDL cholesterol (very low density lipoproteins). These cholesterol particles are rich in triglycerides, which is why individuals with insulin resistance have a high level of triglycerides.

When VLDL particles interact with HDL particles, VLDL exchanges its triglycerides for the cholesterol of HDL particles. This results in a *decrease* in HDL cholesterol. These Triglycerides-enriched HDL particles also break down easily, which lowers HDL level. This is how most Type diabetics with insulin resistance end up with low HDL cholesterol.

HDL cholesterol works as a scavenger by cleansing out the cholesterol deposited in the walls of blood vessels. That is why HDL cholesterol is known as the "good" cholesterol. If your HDL is low, there will be less cleansing of the cholesterol buildup in the vessel wall. Therefore, a low level of HDL cholesterol is a major risk factor for narrowing of coronary blood vessels.

VLDL particles also give rise to the formation of another cholesterol particle known as IDL (intermediate density lipoprotein), which then converts to LDL (low density lipoproteins). VLDL, IDL, and LDL particles deposit in the arterial wall, which causes narrowing of the vessel wall.

**4**. Pattern B LDL Cholesterol Particles

LDL (bad) cholesterol consists of two subpopulations:

• Large, fluffy particles (Pattern A)
• Small, dense particles (Pattern B)

Pattern B particles deposit more easily inside the blood vessel wall compared to  Pattern A particles and, therefore, are more harmful.

In Type 2 diabetic patients with insulin resistance, there is a predominance of the more harmful Pattern B particles, which again leads to narrowing of the coronary blood vessels.

**5**. An Increased Tendency for Clot Formation and Decreased Ability to Break Clots

In Type 2 diabetics with insulin resistance, there is a high level of several clotting factors, including fibrinogen levels in the blood, which increases the risk for blood clot formation.

In addition, these patients also have a decreased ability to break up blood clots. This happens due to a high level of a substance known as PAI–1, short for plasminogen activator inhibitor-1.

Consequently, Type 2 diabetics are at a high risk for blood clot formation and have a decreased ability to break up these clots. When a clot forms in an already narrowed coronary blood vessel, a person might suffer an acute heart attack.

## 6. An Elevated Highly Sensitive CRP (C-Reactive Protein) Level

A high level of C-Reactive Protein indicates ongoing inflammation in the blood vessel wall. Inflammatory cells are present in the atherosclerotic plaque inside the blood vessel wall. When inflamed, these plaques can easily rupture. A ruptured plaque attracts clotting factors. A blood clot forms at the site of a ruptured plaque, which then causes an acute shutdown of blood flow that may result in an acute heart attack.

A high level of CRP, therefore, indicates a significantly higher risk for a heart attack. Type 2 diabetics with insulin resistance usually have a high level of CRP.

## 7. Endothelial Dysfunction

The endothelium, the lining of the blood vessel wall, produces a number of substances, a balance of which is important for its healthy functioning. A number of these substances can cause constriction of the vessel wall (vasoconstriction), while others cause a dilatation of the vessel wall (vasodilatation).

In healthy individuals, there is a fine balance between these two processes. Type 2 diabetics with insulin resistance have a disruption in this balance in such a way that there is *more* vasoconstriction and *less* vasodilatation. This endothelial dysfunction causes further narrowing of the blood vessels.

## Heart Attacks Happen Even After Angioplasty

As all of the above indicates, narrowing of coronary blood vessels is a complex process. It develops over a period of years due to underlying Insulin Resistance Syndrome.

To recap, the process of narrowing of the coronary arteries consists of:

• Deposition of cholesterol in the wall of the coronary arteries

• Proliferation of a variety of cells in the wall of the coronary arteries

• Damage to the lining of the coronary arteries (endothelial dysfunction)

Angioplasty, as well as stent placement, temporarily opens up the narrowed blood vessel, but has no effect on the cholesterol buildup inside the wall of the blood vessel. Hence, after an angioplasty, if appropriate drug therapy is not instituted to treat the disease process inside the wall of the blood vessel, it will shut down again. An angioplasty is a temporary fix. It must be followed by aggressive drug treatment of the underlying disease process.

## Risk For A Heart Attack Even After Bypass Surgery

An acute heart event, such as chest pain, brings patients to the hospital and to the likely diagnosis of a narrowing of the coronary arteries. Usually, they undergo angioplasty, stent placement, and/or heart bypass surgery. These procedures are only temporary solutions to relieve an acute emergency situation and don't treat the underlying cause of the problem: Insulin Resistance Syndrome.

Unfortunately, even at this stage, most patients are not diagnosed with Insulin Resistance Syndrome. Patients think their problem is fixed and they'll be fine as long as they eat right, and take their drugs to lower cholesterol.

As demonstrated above, the process of Insulin Resistance Syndrome and, consequently, narrowing of the blood vessels continues until one day they are again rushed back to the hospital with chest pain only to find they are having another heart attack. Even after heart bypass surgery, it's essential to treat the real cause of narrowing of the coronary arteries — Insulin Resistance Syndrome.

# Chapter 20

# Stroke in Diabetics

A person suffers a stroke when blood flow is cut off from an area of the brain. This results in a neurological symptom, depending on the area of the brain involved.

The usual symptoms of a stroke include weakness in the leg, arm, or an entire side of the body. Sometimes, one side of the face is affected, causing slurred speech, difficulty in swallowing, and deviation of the angle of the mouth to one side. Sometimes, a stroke may cause blurry vision, imbalance, confusion, and even lack of consciousness.

About 50% of stroke survivors live with permanent disabilities such as difficulty in walking, impaired speech, difficulty in self-care, and memory loss. Many stroke survivors visit the hospital numerous times with all sorts of medical problems including frequent pneumonias, recurrent strokes, heart attacks, and bedsores. Most become depressed. Their families also experience physical, emotional, and economic turmoil. Prevention of stroke is the key to this huge medical and psychosocial problem.

Stroke is the third leading cause of death in the United States. The general assumption that stroke is a disease of old age is not a reliable nor an accurate view. A lot of people under the age of sixty-five have strokes. The incidence of stroke more than doubles for each decade after the age of fifty-five.

There are three types of strokes:
- Ischemic strokes
- Embolic strokes

• Hemorrhagic strokes

Ischemic strokes are the most common. These strokes take place when a blood clot forms in an already narrowed blood vessel of the brain. A transient ischemic attack, or TIA, is a minor ischemic stroke.

An embolic stroke occurs when a blood clot forms inside the heart, dislodges, travels to the brain, and blocks a small blood vessel there.

A hemorrhagic stroke occurs when there is bleeding inside the brain.

**Risk For A Stroke**

You are at risk for a stroke if you have any of the following risk factors. The more risk factors you have, the higher the risk of having a stroke.

• Diabetes

• Older than forty-five years old

• Overweight, especially around the waistline. This is also called abdominal obesity (waistline more than 35 inches in women and more than 38 inches in men; among Asians, these numbers are 32 inches for women and 35 inches for men).

• High blood pressure (more than 130/85 mm Hg)

• Low HDL cholesterol (less than 50 mg/dl in females; less than 40 mg/dl in males)

• High triglycerides (more than 150 mg/dl)

• Smoking

• Atrial fibrillation (irregular heart beat)

• Family history of stroke

These risk factors usually don't cause any symptoms. A stroke or a heart attack is usually the first symptom. People want to ignore these risk factors as long as they feel fine. They don't understand that by the time they have symptoms, the quality of their life may never be the same.

Most Type 2 diabetic patients have abdominal obesity, high level of triglycerides, low levels of HDL (good) cholesterol, and high blood pressure. All of these metabolic disorders are major risk factors for a stroke. Again, collectively, these disorders are known as Insulin Resistance Syndrome.

In my practice, I often see middle-aged diabetic patients with high blood pressure. When I tell them they have high blood pressure and need drug therapy, they look surprised and question my diagnosis of hypertension. Sometimes they say, "But my other physician didn't say any thing about it" or "Last month I had it checked at the free screening at the pharmacy and they said it was fine." My favorite line is, "My blood pressure is high because I'm in your office."

Accepting the diagnosis of diabetes, high blood pressure, and cholesterol disorder means that your body is no longer perfect and you must do something about it. Some people take the ostrich approach. They stick their head in the sand and hope it goes away. It's easier to be in denial than to face reality. Diabetes, high blood pressure, and cholesterol disorder need your attention. Don't ignore them.

Strokes are preventable. Early diagnosis and aggressive treatment of the risk factors is the key to the prevention of a stroke. In most Type 2 diabetic patients, a stroke occurs due to narrowing of the blood vessels in the neck and/or in the brain.

Strategies to prevent a stroke in a Type 2 diabetic are the same as in preventing a heart attack, discussed earlier in the previous chapter.

Chapter **21**

# Memory Loss/Dementia in Diabetics

Dementia means a progressive decline in intellectual functioning. Memory loss is a frequent symptom of dementia.

Narrowing of the brain vessels is the underlying cause for intellectual decline and memory loss in a majority of diabetic patients.

Transient ischemic attacks (TIAs), also known as mini-strokes, take place due to transient cessation of blood circulation to a certain part of the brain. Multiple mini-strokes over a period of time lead to the death of brain cells and, eventually, a person starts experiencing a decline in intellectual function and lapses in memory. This is known as multi-infarct dementia or vascular dementia, the most common cause for memory loss in diabetic patients.

Of course, the underlying cause for narrowing of the blood vessels is Insulin Resistance Syndrome. And once again, diabetes, high blood pressure, cholesterol disorder, and abdominal obesity are the main components of Insulin Resistance Syndrome.

In a large clinical study (1), involving 10,963 people, researchers assessed changes in cognitive function over a six-year interval. Diabetes and hypertension were found to be the strongest predictors of decline in intellectual functioning, even as early as at the age of forty-seven.

In another study (2), researchers looked at the impact of ingesting 50 grams of rapidly absorbing carbohydrates (one half of a bagel and white grape juice) on the memory of diabetic patients. They found a positive correlation between carbohydrate intake and poor memory in these patients. In addition, overall poor control of diabetes was associated with a decline in memory.

If you don't aggressively treat the underlying disease that caused a stroke in the first place, how can you prevent further strokes and their consequences, such as memory loss? Quite often, these patients are misdiagnosed with Alzheimer's disease. Another common problem is when patients suffer a heart attack, undergo heart bypass surgery or angioplasty, and they are not properly evaluated or treated for the risk factors for stroke. Remember, if you have narrowing of the blood vessels in your heart, you probably also have narrowing of the blood vessels in your brain, and probably every where in the entire body.

Anyone who has memory loss, a stroke (even a minor stroke), a heart attack, coronary angioplasty, or heart bypass surgery should be evaluated for risk factors for narrowing of the blood vessels.

These risk factors include hypertension, cholesterol disorder, and diabetes or pre-diabetes.

### Other Causes Of Memory Loss/Dementia

Besides vascular dementia, some of the other causes for memory loss or dementia include an underactive thyroid, vitamin B12 deficiency, depression, subdural hematoma, AIDS, and syphilis.

Out of these causes, an underactive thyroid, depression and vitamin B12 deficiency are the most common disorders, which can be easily diagnosed and treated.

A low level of vitamin B12 is common in elderly diabetic individuals who are also on metformin. Vitamin B12 deficiency should be treated either with vitamin B12 injections or with vitamin B12 pills. (See chapter on vitamin B12 deficiency.)

Alzheimer's dementia is a diagnosis of exclusion. That is, once all the treatable causes of dementia as mentioned above have been excluded, only then should a diagnosis of Alzheimer's be made.

## Diagnostic Testing For Memory Loss/Dementia

• Two-hour oral glucose tolerance test to diagnose pre-diabetes or diabetes

• Cholesterol panel, which should include HDL, LDL, and triglycerides

• Ultrasound of carotid arteries to rule out narrowing of the neck arteries

• MRI of the brain to rule out any evidence of a recent or an old stroke

• A thyroid blood panel to diagnose an underactive thyroid

• A blood test for vitamin B12, syphilis, and AIDS

## References

1. Knopman D, et al. Atherosclerosis Risk in Communities (ARIC) cohort.
*Neurology* 2001; 56:42–28.

2. Greenwood CE, Kaplan RJ, et al. Carbohydrate induced memory impairment in adults with type 2 diabetes. *Diabetes Care* 2003; 26:1961–1966.

Chapter **22**

# Kidney Disease In Diabetics

Diabetes is the single largest cause of kidney failure in the U.S., accounting for approximately 40% of all cases. These patients then require chronic dialysis or a kidney transplant to stay alive.

It's estimated that kidney failure requiring dialysis will develop in 20% to 40% of Type 2 diabetics who have diabetes for more than ten years. By the year 2020, it's estimated that 80% of dialysis patients will be Type 2 diabetics.

Diabetes, along with high blood pressure, affects kidney function slowly over a period of years. You don't develop symptoms due to diabetic kidney disease until it is too late and you're about to go on dialysis. Remember, diabetes is a silent killer.

### Misconceptions About Chronic Kidney Disease

- Often people have the misconception that if you're urinating fine, then your kidney must be functioning normally. Wrong! You will continue to urinate without symptoms while diabetes and high blood pressure damage your kidneys. Pain, burning, or difficulty urinating are usually symptoms of urinary bladder infection or prostate enlargement, not kidney disease.

- People often mistakenly think that pain in the lumber region is due to kidney disease. Pain in the lumbar region is almost always due to diseases of the lumbar spine, such as a herniated disc, arthritis, or a muscle spasm.

Only rarely are kidneys responsible for pain in the lumber region.

- Another misconception is that if your kidney ultrasound or CT scan is normal, then your kidneys must be normal, too. The fact is that these imaging tests focus on structural problems in the kidneys, such as stone formation, obstruction or tumors. Diabetes and high blood pressure, on the other hand, cause a chronic, slow decline in kidney function. Diabetic kidney disease is diagnosed by utilizing blood and urine tests.

Before I discuss how diabetes affects your kidneys, let me first briefly explain what are the normal functions of the kidneys.

## Normal Functions Of The Kidneys

By far, the most important function of the kidneys is to form urine and, thereby, remove waste products of cellular metabolism from the blood stream and deposit them into the urine.

The basic functioning unit of the kidneys is called the nephron. The formation of urine takes place in the nephron as a result of filtration of water, electrolytes (such as sodium, potassium, and calcium), and waste products of metabolism (such as creatinine from the muscles).

Clinically, the filtration rate of the kidneys is called GFR (Glomerular Filtration Rate). It is measured as creatinine clearance, a test that involves collecting urine for a twenty-four-hour period. Blood urea nitrogen (BUN) and serum creatinine are the typical tests for kidney function and are included in most blood chemistry panels. Serum creatinine is a more accurate test for kidney function than BUN. In the US, laboratories use serum creatinine and give an estimated GFR.

## The Other Important Functions Of The Kidneys:

• Regulation of electrolytes (such as potassium, sodium, and calcium) in the blood

- Maintaining adequate hydration

- Regulation of blood pressure

- Regulation of vitamin D metabolism

- Production of a hormone, erythropoietin, which is important for the normal production of red blood cells

## Stages In The Development Of Diabetic Kidney Disease

Diabetes affects kidneys slowly over a period of years and causes a progressive decrease in kidney functions. We divide this gradual decline in kidney functions into five stages.

### *Stage 1: Hyperfiltration*

There is an increase in the filtration rate at the nephron level, which is the basic functioning unit of the kidney.

Normal creatinine clearance is 80–120 ml/minute. In the stage of hyperfiltration, the creatinine clearance rate may be as high as 170 ml/minute or more. In the blood chemistry panel, BUN and creatinine are normal at this stage. Patients do not have any symptoms at this stage of diabetic kidney disease, which usually lasts several years.

Diabetic kidney disease is easily halted and even reversed at this point. Therefore, it is very important to diagnose kidney disease at this stage. This can easily be accomplished by measuring creatinine clearance, which requires a twenty-four-hour urine collection.

### *Stage 2: Microalbuminuria*

At this stage, albumin, a special protein, starts to leak into the urine due to damage to the wall of the nephron. Clinically, this albumin leakage can be detected by measuring albumin excretion in the urine. A urinary albumin excretion of more than 30 mg but less than 300 mg in a twenty-four-hour period is known as microalbuminuria. In the blood chemistry panel, BUN and creatinine are usually normal at this stage.

As with Stage 1 diabetic kidney disease, patients do not have any symptoms of diabetic kidney disease at this stage, which usually lasts for several years.

Routine urine testing does not detect this small amount of albumin excretion. Instead, three special methods of screening for microalbumin excretion are available:

- Measurement of albumin-to-creatinine ratio in a random urine sample
- Timed (four hours or overnight) urine collection
- Twenty-four-hour urine collection

Diabetic kidney disease at this stage can be halted and even reversed in a majority of patients.

## Stage 3: Frank Proteinuria

With further progression of diabetic kidney disease, larger quantities of albumin start to spill into the urine. If a twenty-four hour urine albumin excretion exceeds 300 mg in twenty-four hours, it is called frank proteinuria. In the blood chemistry panel, BUN and creatinine may be abnormal at this stage. This stage of diabetic kidney disease may last a few years.

Patients in this stage may start experiencing some ankle swelling. Many patients, however, do not experience any symptoms at this stage.

## Stage 4: Nephrotic Syndrome

With further progression of diabetic kidney disease, urinary protein excretion may reach several thousand milligrams per day. A proteinuria of more than 3000 mg in twenty-four hours is known as nephrotic range proteinuria. In the blood chemistry panel, BUN and creatinine are usually abnormal at this stage.

Often patients have high blood pressure as well. Patients with nephrotic syndrome usually have symptoms of leg swelling, abdominal swelling, and even shortness of breath, due to the accumulation of fluid inside the chest cavity.

## Stage 5: End Stage Renal Disease

In this stage, patients have many symptoms such as fatigue, leg swelling, poor appetite, intractable itching, and mental confusion.

In the blood chemistry panel, BUN and creatinine are always abnormal at this stage. Patients also have high blood pressure, which is usually difficult to treat.

These patients are treated with chronic dialysis, usually three times a week. They are prone to all sorts of complications, such as infections and clotting of the dialysis access, low blood counts, high risk for bleeding, vitamin D deficiency, parathyroid disease, and osteoporosis. These patients are also at a very high risk for heart attacks, strokes, and leg amputations. They are usually frequent visitors to the hospital. Quality of life is often poor at this stage.

## Preventing Kidney Disease

Fortunately, diabetic kidney disease can be prevented, but only with early diagnosis and aggressive treatment of diabetes and high blood pressure. Unfortunately, diabetes and hypertension remain undiagnosed and untreated in millions of people worldwide.

By the time diabetes is diagnosed, a number of people have already developed diabetic kidney disease. Several excellent clinical studies, including my own clinical experience, have demonstrated that aggressive control of blood glucose and high blood pressure can significantly reduce the risk for kidney disease.

By using the five-step treatment approach, I have been able to prevent end stage renal disease in the vast majority of my diabetic patients.

## Recommendations To Prevent Kidney Failure In Diabetics

### 1. Good Control of Diabetes

Kidney disease primarily develops in those patients who have poor control of diabetes. Excellent control of diabetes can prevent development of kidney disease.

I set the following targets for controlling diabetes in my patients.

*Target Blood Glucose Values*

• Premeal blood glucose levels should be 90–120 mg/dl.
• Two-hour postmeal blood glucose levels should be less than 140 mg/dl
• Hemoglobin A1c (HbA1c) should be less than 6.0%

### 2. Good Control of Blood Pressure

Hypertension should be aggressively treated in diabetic patients. I aim for blood pressure to be less than 130/80 mm Hg in most of my diabetic patients.

The selection of drugs to control blood pressure is important.

I use ACE(Angiotensin Converting Enzyme) inhibitors and/or ARB (Angiotensin Receptor Blocking) drugs as the first choice to treat high blood pressure in diabetic patients. Several excellent scientific studies have clearly demonstrated that the ACE inhibitors as well as ARBs *not* only control high blood pressure, but also preserve kidney function.

Other drugs that can be used to treat severe high blood pressure include:

• Diuretics, in small doses (such as hydrochlorthiazide or indapamide)

- Calcium channel blockers (such as Norvasc, diltiazem, or verapamil)
- Alpha blockers (such as Cardura)
- Beta-blockers (such as carvedilol, atenolol or metoprolol)
- Centrally acting drugs such as clonidine

### 3. Urinary Microalbumin Excretion Test

This special urine test should be done on a yearly basis, especially if your diabetes is not optimally controlled.

A routine urine test does not check for it. As I mentioned earlier, there are three ways to carry out this test.
- Measurement of albumin-to-creatinine ratio in a random urine sample
- Timed (four hours or overnight) urine collection
- Twenty-four-hour urine collection

Diabetic patients who have microalbuminuria should be considered for an ACE inhibitor or an angiotensin receptor blocking (ARB) drug even if their blood pressure is not elevated, only if they don't develop symptoms of low blood pressure.

A number of well-designed scientific studies have shown that ACE (Angiotensin Converting Enzyme) inhibitors as well as ARB (Angiotensin Receptor Blocking) drugs can reduce microalbuminuria and slow down the progression of diabetic kidney disease.

But I must emphasize that an excellent control of diabetes is the most important factor to prevent as well slow down chronic kidney disease in diabetics. The case of Susan (Case Study #5 from Chapter on Treatment of Diabetes) is a good example. She was on an ARB drug, Losartan, but she was still having marked albuminuria, as her diabetes was uncontrolled. Once, her diabetes got under better control, her albuminria reduced markedly within a matter of few months.

## ACE (Angiotensin Converting Enzyme) Inhibitors

| Brand Name | Generic Name |
|---|---|
| Altace | Ramipril |
| Accupril | Quinapril |
| Lotensin | Benazepril |
| Monopril | Fosinopril |
| Zestril/ Prinivil | Lisinopril |
| Aceon | Perindopril |
| Vasotec | Enalapril |
| Capoten | Captopril |

## ARB (Angiotensin Receptor Blocking) Drugs

| Brand Name | Generic Name |
|---|---|
| Diovan | Valsartan |
| Cozaar | Losartan |
| Avapro | Irbesartan |
| Atacand | Candesartan |
| Micardis | Telmisartan |
| Benicar | Olmesartan |

Here is another case study from my practice to illustrate these points.

# Case Study # 6

Betsy, a fifty five-year-old Caucasian female came to see me with Type 2 diabetes that had been diagnosed ten years before I met her.

Initially, she was on various sulfonylurea drugs (Micronase, Diabeta, Glucotrol) for a few years. Later, she was switched to insulin therapy as sulfonylurea drugs failed to control her diabetes.

At the time I saw her, she was on NPH insulin 40 units plus Regular insulin 20 units, in the morning and in the evening. In addition to diabetes, she had cholesterol disorder, obesity, and high blood pressure. During this time, she also had developed heart disease, breast cancer, and peripheral neuropathy of her feet—all complications of insulin resistance.

## Medications

NPH insulin 40 units plus Regular insulin 20 units, in the morning and in the evening
Aspirin,
Cardizem CD 120 mg twice a day
Lopid 600 mg twice a day

## Physical Examination

Blood Pressure = 110/70 mm Hg
Weight = 208 lbs
Height = 5'5" (about 70 lbs overweight)
Vibration sense decreased in both feet
Rest of the examination was unremarkable

## Laboratory Results

Fasting blood glucose = 167 mg/dl

HbA1c = 8.6%

Triglycerides = 353 mg/dl

HDL Cholesterol = 27 mg/dl

LDL Cholesterol = 187 mg/dl

## Diagnosis

Betsy suffered from Insulin Resistance Syndrome, manifesting as diabetes, high blood pressure, high triglycerides, low HDL, and obesity. Her LDL cholesterol was also elevated.

She had developed coronary heart disease, breast cancer, and peripheral neuropathy as complications of insulin resistance and diabetes.

A twenty-four hour urinary albumin excretion turned out to be markedly elevated at **776 mg** (should be less than 25 mg), indicating she had also developed significant kidney disease due to uncontrolled diabetes. She was on her way to kidney dialysis.

## Treatment

I discussed my 5-step treatment with Betsy in length. Gradually, I took her off insulin and placed her on oral drugs. Her diabetes and blood pressure have remained under pretty good control over the past 11 years.

Betsy had developed significant diabetic kidney disease as evidenced by marked urinary albumin excretion of **776** mg in twenty-four hours (normal being less than 25 mg). Fortunately, we were able to normalize her urinary albumin excretion by employing my 5-step treatment strategy that focuses on aggressive control of insulin resistance.

Her serum creatinine - a measure of kidney function- has also stayed normal over these years.

## Kidney Progress Report

|  | Initial | 6 Months | 11 Months | 31 Months | 10 years | 11 years |
|---|---|---|---|---|---|---|
| 24-hour Urinary Albumin Excretion  (In mg) | 776 | 432 | 420 | 15 | 124 | 63 |
| *Serum Cr  (In mg/dL) | 0.8 | 1.0 | 0.9 | 0.8 | 0.7 | 0.7 |

*Serum Creatinine = Normal range 0.6 - 1.3  mg/dL

In addition, Betsy has not developed any symptoms of coronary artery disease over the past eleven years.

In conclusion, you can effectively reverse your diabetic nephropathy with excellent control of your insulin resistance and Type 2 diabetes. In this way, you can also stop the progression of your coronary artery disease.

Chapter **23**

# Diabetic Peripheral Neuropathy

Diabetic peripheral neuropathy usually causes symptoms such as tingling, a pins-and-needles sensation, a burning sensation, numbness, or pain. Symptoms are usually worse at night and can interfere with sleep. Initially, it affects the toes, which progresses to the entire foot and eventually can progress to the entire lower leg. Later in the course of the disease, hands can also be involved.

Numb feet are at a high risk for injury, such as by accidental scalding from hot water or by accidental puncture, like a small piece of gravel into the sole of the foot. Because of a lack of sensation, wounds go unnoticed, especially in between the toes and on the soles of the feet. Infection settles in these wounds and can cause serious destruction to soft tissues and even extend to the underlying bone. Bone infection is very difficult to treat and may require amputation and a prolonged course of antibiotics.

Early diagnosis is important in order to prevent further progression of this complication. An endocrinologist and a neurologist can diagnose peripheral neuropathy at an early stage. Often, it requires specialized diagnostic testing.

Peripheral neuropathy often starts years before a person is diagnosed with diabetes. An oral glucose tolerance test (OGTT) can diagnose diabetes as well as pre-diabetes many years earlier.

Other factors that can contribute toward peripheral neuropathy:

• Vitamin B12 deficiency, which is common in those on metformin

• Excessive alcohol use

• Vitamin D, calcium, potassium, and magnesium deficiencies often mimic symptoms of peripheral neuropathy. Vitamin D deficiency is extremely commonly, especially in elderly patients as well as in individuals who avoid sun exposure. Potassium and magnesium deficiencies are frequently present in patients who are on diuretics.

## Prevention Is The Best Treatment

Good blood glucose control can prevent the development of peripheral neuropathy. Therefore, excellent blood glucose control is crucial right from the time of the diagnosis of diabetes.

# Treatment Options for Peripheral Neuropathy

Again, good control of diabetes using my five-step treatment strategy is crucial, as it prevents further progression of neuropathy.

A spouse or a friend should regularly examine your feet for any ulcer or sign of infection. See a podiatrist on a regular basis.

There are also some vitamin therapies and prescription medications that can help reduce the symptoms of peripheral neuropathy.

### 1. Alpha-Lipoic Acid

As discussed in Chapter 13 , alpha-lipoic acid is a dietary supplement that has been used in Germany for more than thirty years for the treatment of diabetic neuropathy.

As I mentioned earlier, several clinical studies have shown the effectiveness of alpha-lipoic acid in treating peripheral neuropathy.

I use alpha-lipoic acid in my diabetic patients with peripheral neuropathy and have seen some good results. I feel that this product is safe. I have not seen any serious side effects in my patients. The usual dose is 600–1200 mg/day.

## 2. Capsaicin

For superficial, burning-type pain, capsaicin works pretty well. It is a skin cream that is applied to the affected area, usually the feet. Capsaicin is derived from hot red peppers.
It takes about two to three weeks before the pain starts subsiding. Beware! Initially it may cause some worsening of pain.

## 3. Cymbalta (Duloxetine)

In 2004, the drug Cymbalta was approved for the treatment of diabetic peripheral neuropathy. It works well in about 60% of patients. Most common side effects include dry mouth, nausea, constipation, diarrhea, dizziness, and hot flashes. Cymbalta is also used to treat depression.

## 4. Neurontin (Gabapentin)

Neurontin is an anti-seizure drug that is often used to treat the pain of peripheral neuropathy. Most patients tolerate this drug fairly well. Drowsiness, dizziness, and fatigue are the typical complaints I have heard from patients who are on this medication, especially at higher doses.

On rare occasions, other seizure medications such as Dilantin (phenytoin) and Tegretol (carbamazepine) are used to treat diabetic peripheral neuropathy. These drugs have serious side effects and should only be prescribed by a physician knowledgeable about these drugs.

## 5. Nortriptyline, Amitriptyline, Desipramine.

These are older anti-depression drugs that have been used to treat the pain of peripheral neuropathy. Patients often do not tolerate these drugs well due to their common side effects, which include drowsiness, dizziness, dry mouth, impotence, retention of urine, and heart arrhythmias. These drugs *must not* be used in patients with a history of glaucoma, urinary retention, and heart arrhythmias.

## 6. Mexitil (Mexiletine)

Mexitil is a heart medicine used to treat arrhythmia. It has also been used to treat diabetic peripheral neuropathy. Due to its potential serious side effects, this drug should only be prescribed by a physician experienced in prescribing this drug, such as a cardiologist.

# Case Study #7

Steve, a thirty-seven-year-old Caucasian male, developed symptoms of excruciating pain in his feet, excessive urination, and excessive thirst about six months prior to seeing me.

After testing, he was found to have a markedly elevated blood glucose level of 294 mg/dl and was diagnosed with diabetes. His primary care physician started him on Glucovance 1.25/250 a day (Glucovance is a combination of glyburide and metformin). Then he was referred to me for further management.

### *Physical Examination*

Blood pressure = 135/95 mm Hg
Weight = 206 lbs (about 25 lbs overweight)

### *Laboratory Results*

Fasting blood glucose = 273 mg/dl

Hemoglobin A1c = 11.7%

Triglycerides = 150 mg/dl

HDL cholesterol = 34 mg/dl

LDL cholesterol = 127 mg/dl

## Diagnosis

I diagnosed Steve with Insulin Resistance Syndrome consisting of diabetes, high blood pressure, and low HDL cholesterol. I suspected that the pain in his feet was due to diabetic peripheral neuropathy. I also referred Steve to a neurologist for further diagnostic testing and treatment of his peripheral neuropathy.

## Treatment

Steve and I discussed my five-step approach in length.

### 1. Diabetes Control

Within two months, his diabetes came under excellent control. Steve has maintained excellent control of his diabetes over the twelve years he has been under my care.

### Diabetes Progress Report

|  | Initial | 2 months | 2 years | 4 years | 6 years | 8 years | 10 years | 12 years |
|---|---|---|---|---|---|---|---|---|
| FBG | 273 | 98 | 98 | 102 | 95 | 95 | 87 | 111 |
| HbA1c | 11.7 | 5.9 | 5.2 | 5.1 | 5.6 | 5.5 | 5.4 | 5.6 |

*FBG = Fasting Blood Glucose in mg/dl*
*HbA1c = Hemoglobin A1c in %*

## 2. Peripheral Neuropathy

Steve was started on Neurontin 300 mg/day, which was gradually increased over several months to 600 mg four times a day to control his disabling pain. It took many months before his excruciating pain started to improve. Later, I added alpha-lipoic acid, which helped to bring the dose of Neurontin down to 600 mg two times a day. On this regimen, his pain of neuropathy is under good control.

At four years after his initial diagnosis, his neurologist repeated his nerve conduction study and was truly amazed to find out that not only did Steve's neuropathy not worsen (as is the usual course), but it had also markedly improved. It has remained stable at this improved state over all these years.

This reversal of diabetic peripheral neuropathy is unheard of in medical literature. For me, nothing is more rewarding than to see results like this in my patients. Steve is very pleased with the progress he has made.

## 3. Hypertension

A prescription for Altace 2.5 mg/day nicely controlled Steve's high blood pressure over ten years. Two years ago, Altace was discontinued as he developed an allergy to it. Since then, he is maintaining excellent blood pressure without any medications.

**In summary, you can prevent the development of peripheral neuropathy in the first place. After you develop peripheral neuropathy, you can control it effectively. You can even reverse it. Excellent control of diabetes is the key.**

Chapter **24**

# Diabetic
# Autonomic Neuropathy

The autonomic nervous system controls the function of our various organs such as the heart, stomach, intestine, urinary bladder, and, in men, the penis. Diabetes often affects this autonomic nervous system and can cause the following symptoms:

• Fullness and bloating in the upper abdomen after eating. This happens due to the slowing of stomach emptying. Technically, this condition is known as diabetic gastroparesis.

• Chronic diarrhea

• Chronic constipation

• Impotence

• Urinary incontinence

• Dizziness upon standing due to a drop in blood pressure

• Excessive sweating

• Heart arrhythmia (excessively fast or slow heart rate)

Physicians often forget to think of diabetic autonomic neuropathy as a cause of these symptoms. As a result, patients usually undergo an extensive diagnostic workup that does not accurately diagnose their problem. Patients often undergo procedures such as CT scans, MRI scans, colonoscopies, and gastroscopies. These procedures might detect anatomic problems, but autonomic neuropathy affects the function of an organ, and, therefore, does not show up on these tests.

An experienced endocrinologist is your best bet in diagnosing these disorders correctly. Most of these disorders are diagnosed clinically and require the clinical skills of an endocrinologist.

Some specialized tests are used to confirm the clinical diagnosis of autonomic dysfunction. A special nuclear scan test that involves a test-meal, can accurately assess the emptying of the stomach and, therefore, diagnose diabetic gastroparesis. Autonomic neuropathy of the heart can be diagnosed with a test known as the heart rate variability test.

### Treatment of Diabetic Autonomic Neuropathy

Good control of diabetes can prevent further progression of the problems associated with diabetic autonomic neuropathy. Therefore, aim for excellent control of diabetes, targeting your hemoglobin A1c to be less than 6.0%.

Each of these conditions should be properly diagnosed by an experienced physician and treated accordingly.

Chapter **25**

# Impotence in Diabetics

Impotence is common among diabetics. However, impotence can be due to a variety of reasons other than diabetes and, therefore, should be thoroughly evaluated by an expert in this field, preferably an endocrinologist.

Various causes of impotence include:

• Autonomic neuropathy due to uncontrolled diabetes

• Poor circulation due to diabetes and Insulin Resistance Syndrome

• Smoking

• Excessive alcohol consumption

• Certain drugs such as beta-blockers, thiazide diuretics, spironolactone, clonidine, antidepressants, anti-anxiety drugs, cimetidine, ranitidine, metoclopramide, and soy products

• Low testosterone level

• High prolactin level, a hormone produced by the pituitary gland

• Prostate surgery

• Psychological problems

In most diabetic patients, impotence is a complex problem. There are *multiple* factors working in concert that lead to impotence.

- Usually, diabetes is uncontrolled

- The patient is not on insulin-sensitizing drugs, which are Actos, and metformin

- The patient is on beta-blockers to control hypertension

- HDL cholesterol is low and triglycerides are high

- Circulation is poor

- The patient feels quite tired all the time due to a variety of reasons including uncontrolled diabetes, obesity, side effects of medicines, lack of vitamin D and other vitamins and minerals, and the stress of daily life. You are not interested in sex when you're tired, fatigued and stressed out

- Often these patients are depressed. Having sex is the last thing on their mind

## Treatment Of Impotence

Treatment of impotence is quite challenging. My approach to the treatment of impotence in diabetic patients is as follows:

- First, I thoroughly evaluate a patient for all of the causes mentioned above

- I treat all the factors that I can identify in an individual patient

- I treat their diabetes as well as other components of Insulin Resistance Syndrome, such as hypertension and cholesterol disorder, aggressively with my 5-step treatment approach

- I try to stop any medicines that may contribute to impotence, such as beta-blockers, spironolactone, metoclopramide, or soy products

- I make sure prolactin is not elevated and testosterone levels are normal for the patient's age

• I strongly encourage smokers to quit smoking

• Those who are overweight are encouraged to lose weight, which also helps increase energy

• With proper amounts of vitamin D, calcium, potassium, magnesium, and other mineral supplements, they start feeling better

• I also address their depression with my stress management strategy.

After correcting all of these factors, I sometimes prescribe drugs such as Viagra, Cialis, or Levitra

## Viagra

Viagra must be taken about an hour before sexual activity. Headache, flushing, and dizziness are frequent complaints that I have heard from my patients using Viagra.

Please note that Viagra use has caused several deaths. Therefore, you should be very careful about using this drug. Patients on nitrates and alpha blockers such as Cardura (doxazosin), Hytrin (terazosin) must not use Viagra. Patients with heart disease should check with their cardiologist before using Viagra.

## Cialis and Levitra

After Viagra, two other drugs called Cialis and Levitra were released in the U.S. for treatment of impotence. These are in the same class of drugs as Viagra. Their onset of action is faster than Viagra.

Cialis is effective during a twenty-four-hour period after its intake. Therefore, you have more flexibility about the timing of your sexual activity. Side effects of both Cialis and Levitra are similar to side effects of Viagra.

## Other Options

Other older treatment options for impotence include a vacuum pump, injection of Caverject into the penis, MUSE, and lastly, a penile implant.

*A vacuum pump* works for some patients. Patients taking blood thinners should avoid it. A vacuum pump may cause bruising of the penis.

*With Caverject* a special chemical known as prostaglandin E1 is delivered by injection into the penis. You need to learn the injection technique from a nurse at a urologist's office. Penile pain and excessive stimulation of the penis are the main problems with these injections. However, it works in most people with impotence.

*With MUSE (Medicated Urethral System for Erection)*, prostaglandin E1 is delivered through the opening at the tip of the penis. Penile pain, excessive stimulation of the penis, and dizziness are the main problems with this technique. It works in about 50% of patients with impotence.

*A penile implant* should be the last resort. It involves surgery that has its own complications.

Chapter **26**

# Poor Circulation in the Legs in Diabetics

Diabetics frequently have poor circulation in their legs, which can eventually lead to amputation. The typical symptom of poor circulation is pain in the legs, especially while walking, that subsides upon resting. In severe cases, this pain is present even at rest.

Poor circulation develops due to narrowing of the arterial blood vessels, a complication of Insulin Resistance Syndrome. Narrowing of blood vessels is a generalized process affecting all arterial blood vessels in the body. If you have blockages of the coronary arteries in your heart, you may also have blockages in the arterial blood vessels in your legs, brain and intestines.

I often see patients who have undergone angioplasty of their heart arteries but are totally unaware that they may also have poor circulation in their legs.

### Diagnostic Testing For Poor Circulation In The Legs

You should have a Doppler ultrasound test of your leg arteries if you have symptoms of poor circulation. This is a simple, noninvasive, outpatient test that can easily diagnose peripheral arterial disease in the legs.

In most patients, treatment is with medications and no further testing is required. In patients with severe peripheral arterial disease, angioplasty or surgery is sometimes required. In these patients, an angiogram of the leg arteries is done prior to an angioplasty or surgery.

## Treatment

Prevention is the best treatment. Early diagnosis and appropriate treatment of diabetes can prevent this devastating complication of diabetes. With my five-step treatment approach to diabetes, I have been able to prevent leg amputation in the vast majority of my patients.

Once you've developed poor circulation in your legs, aggressive control of diabetes and other components of Insulin Resistance Syndrome with appropriate drugs can prevent further progression of this disease and may save your limbs.

Patients who smoke cigarettes are putting fuel on the fire. Smokers *must* quit smoking in order to prevent leg amputation.

Certain drugs such as Trental (pentoxifylline) and Pletal (cilostazol) may somewhat help in the treatment of poor circulation.

Chapter **27**

# Eye Disease in Diabetics

Diabetes gradually affects eyes over a period of years. It affects the innermost layer of the eye, known as the retina. Hence, the condition is known as diabetic retinopathy.

Diabetes is the leading cause of blindness in the U.S. Fortunately, this debilitating condition can be prevented by aggressive treatment of diabetes right from the start.

At the Jamila Diabetes & Endocrine Medical Center, I have been able to prevent diabetic retinopathy in the vast majority of my patients.

Outline of My approach to Prevent/Treat Diabetic retinopathy includes:

*1. Aggressive Control of Blood Glucose in Most Type 2 Diabetic Patients, but without the risk of Hypoglycemia.*

Therefore, I avoid insulin in my Type 2 diabetics, which is the most common cause of hypoglycemia.

Using my 5-step approach, I aim for a HbA1c less than 6.0%.

*2. Aggressive Control of High Blood Pressure*

Hypertension occurs much more frequently in patients with diabetes. Hypertension itself can cause eye damage. Therefore, the combination of hypertension and diabetes is very detrimental for eyes.

Blood pressure should be less than 130/85 mm Hg in a diabetic patient.

Chapter **28**

# Fatty Liver in Diabetics

Uncontrolled diabetes can also affect your liver. This condition is known as fatty liver. In medical terms, it is called NAFLD (Non-Alcoholic Fatty Liver Disease), which simply means increased deposition of fat in your liver. Sometimes, this condition can lead to inflammation of the liver cells, which is called NASH (Non-Alcoholic Steato-Hepatitis). Often, you don't have any symptoms due to this condition. However, in some cases it can lead to cirrhosis of the liver, which is a very serious disease that can be fatal.

In most patients, NAFLD/NASH results from abnormal fat metabolism in the liver due to underlying insulin resistance. Obesity and in particular abdominal obesity seems to play a central role in causing NAFLD/NASH. Insulin resistance in fat cells leads to increased breakdown of fat, which causes an increased flux of free fatty acids into the liver. High insulin level, which is present in these patients with insulin resistance, promotes increased synthesis of fat from free fatty acids in the liver. As a result, there is an increased accumulation of fat in liver cells.

In addition, oxidative stress, which is common in the presence of insulin resistance, can initiate cell death and scarring inside the liver. Therefore, in any individual with clinical features of insulin resistance syndrome and an abnormal liver function test, NASH should be on top of the list of possible diagnosis.

## Diagnosis Of Fatty Liver

There are no established standards for screening with imaging studies for NAFLD/NASH.

Ultrasound can detect moderate to severe fat accumulation in liver, but fails to detect fatty liver if fat accumulation is less than 18 %. Ultrasound of the liver can be difficult in these patients who are often obese. Also, it cannot distinguish between simple fatty liver (NAFLD) and NASH. In the same way, a CT scan can diagnose moderate to severe fat accumulation in the liver, but the scan can be normal in mild cases.

A new technology called MR spectroscopy (Magnetic Resonance Spectroscopy) appears to be a promising imaging modality, but is available at only a few academic institutions and is expensive. Liver biopsy is supposedly the gold-standard method, but it is invasive, costly and impractical considering the vast number of patients afflicted with NAFLD. Even when liver biopsy is performed, a single core biopsy is of lower diagnostic yield compared to multiple core biopsies.

## My Practical Approach To Diagnose NASH

Since 2000, we have been carefully investigating abnormal liver enzymes in patients with any <u>2</u> of the following features of Insulin Resistance Syndrome :

- Abdominal obesity (BMI > 25)
- Hypertension (BP > 130/85 mm Hg)
- Elevated serum triglycerides > 150 mg/dl.
- Low HDL ( < 40 mg/dl in male, < 50 mg/dl in female)
- Pre-diabetes (fasting blood glucose 100-125 mg/dl {Impaired Fasting Glucose, IFG} or 2-hr blood. glucose > 140 mg/dl in 2-hr OGTT { Impaired Glucose Tolerance, IGT}.
- Type 2 diabetes, fasting blood glucose equal or more than 126 mg/dl.

Criteria for the diagnosis of NASH:

In patients with Insulin Resistance Syndrome, we decided to use the following clinical parameters to identify patients with NASH.

- Presence of at least 2 of the features of Insulin Resistance Syndrome.
- Elevated ALT more than 45 U/L
- Use of alcohol limited to no more than 2 drinks (about 20 g) per day.
- Negative serology for Hepatitis A, B, and C .
- Absence of a drug known to cause liver injury.

ALT (alanine aminotransferase), AST (aspartate aminotransferase), bilirubin, and albumin are blood tests for liver function, and are included in most blood chemistry panels. Elevation in ALT and AST is usually the first indication of liver disease including fatty liver. In more advanced cases of liver disease, serum bilirubin gets elevated, and serum albumin goes down.

The most common causes for abnormal liver function include fatty liver, drugs, alcoholism, and hepatitis. Your physician needs to carefully look into these common causes for abnormal liver function.

## Treatment Of Fatty Liver (NAFLD and NASH)

Treatment of NASH is in the rudimentary stages.

I believe that treatment of NASH should focus on treating its cause, insulin resistance, which requires a comprehensive approach. Insulin resistance is caused by five factors: genetics, aging, abdominal obesity, sedentary life-style and stress. Therefore, I utilize my 5-step approach, described earlier, to treat insulin resistance in my Type 2 diabetic patients with fatty liver. With this approach, I have seen good results in my patients with fatty liver disease.

In a placebo-controlled study (1), Actos (pioglitazone) was shown to be effective and safe in treating biopsy-proven NASH patients who also had pre-diabetes or Type 2 diabetes. Metformin has been studied mostly in small uncontrolled trials. In one small study (2), researchers noticed some beneficial effects of metformin on fatty liver disease.

## References

1. Belfort R[1], Harrison SA, Brown K, Darland C, Finch J, Hardies J, Balas B, Gastaldelli A, Tio F, Pulcini J, Berria R, Ma JZ, Dwivedi S, Havranek R, Fincke C, DeFronzo R, Bannayan GA, Schenker S, Cusi K. A placebo-controlled trial of pioglitazone in subjects with nonalcoholic steatohepatitis. *N Engl J Med.* 2006 Nov 30;355(22):2297-307.

2. Marchesini G, Brizi M, Bianchi G, Tomassetti S, Zoli M, Melchionda N. Metformin in non-alcoholic steatohepatitis. *Lancet.* 2001 Sep 15;358(9285):893-4.

Chapter **29**

# Decreased Immunity Against Infections in Diabetics

Diabetics are more susceptible to infections. Skin infections are rather common among diabetics and take longer to heal. Other infections include urinary tract infections, upper respiratory infections and pneumonias.

If your diabetes is uncontrolled, your immune system cannot fight off infections effectively. High blood glucose itself weakens your immune system. In addition, uncontrolled diabetes also frequently leads to poor circulation, especially in the legs. Because of poor circulation, your immune cells have difficulty reaching the infected area of the skin. That's why a skin wound, which would heal up in a non-diabetic person without any problems, may become a non-healing wound in a diabetic person which sometimes ends up in an amputation of the toe, foot or even a leg.

In addition, diabetics are particularly low in vitamin D. Modern research has clearly established that vitamin D plays a vital role in the *normal* functioning of the Immune System. In response to an invading pathogen such as a virus or a bacterium, vitamin D helps immune cells to produce a number of antimicrobial chemicals, in particular a chemical called **cathelicidin antimicrobial peptide** (CAMP), which works like an antibiotic, but without the side-effects associated with antibiotics. Therefore, if you are low in vitamin D, you have an increased susceptibility to all sorts of infections.

Diabetics are also low in Zinc, as I mentioned earlier in the book, which is an important mineral that helps us to fight off infections.

**Here are some helpful tips to fight off infections:**

- Maintain good nutrition, as outlined earlier in the book.

- Take Vitamin D on a regular basis. Have your Vitamin D level checked every 3 - 4 months to make sure that you have a good level of vitamin D. If you develop any infection, double the dose of vitamin D until your infection clears up.

- Take good care of your diabetes. Aim for good control of your blood glucose while being careful to avoid hypoglycemia. Good control of blood glucose helps to improve your immune function.

- Stress wreaks havoc on our immune system. Stress management should become part of your daily routine. Please refer to the chapter on stress management.

- Take common sense precautions to avoid infections. For example, never walk barefoot. This may prevent any small, dirty, sharp object from penetrating the bottom of your foot. This may end up saving your limb.

- Take any infection seriously. Notify your doctor promptly and seek advice.

- For superficial, localized skin wounds, I utilize Hydrogen Peroxide and/or Betadine for local wound care in my Type 2 diabetic patients.

- For an ongoing infection you need an antibiotic.

# Recipes

# Recipes

This section contains a number of my original recipes. Sounds shocking! A doctor talking about recipes. I understand your shock.

Let me share my own journey regarding cooking. Until the age of about 35, I did not know much about cooking. My cooking skills were limited to making a cup of tea, an omelet and toast. Then, my mother came to live with me, as she had become disabled due to a stroke. Back then, there was no Indian restaurant in my town. As a necessity, I started cooking at home, because she did not care for regular American food. As I would cook, my mother would also be in the kitchen in her wheelchair, giving instructions, step by step. The results were pretty good. It encouraged me and I started to like cooking.

As an endocrinologist, I realized the important role food plays in our health. I clearly see we are what we eat. Gradually, I got more and more involved in cooking. I did not follow any cook books. I simply followed the basic principles of Indian cooking I learned from my mother and improvised my own recipes.

Now, I love cooking. With the help of my lovely wife, we even grow our own vegetables, herbs and fruits. We also have our own chickens. They are great pets because they lay eggs, keep the yard fertilized, eat snails and children love them. You don't have to have a rooster for hens to lay eggs, a fact many people don't know.

It is such a pleasure to just walk into the back yard and pick fresh vegetables and herbs. While cooking breakfast, I bath in the morning sun, while doing yoga and meditation at the same time. Actually, cooking keeps you in the Now and whenever you are in the Now, you are meditating. The purpose of meditation is to shift your attention into the Now.

Each and every one of these recipes has been subjected to the taste buds of my wife and some friends. I hope you enjoy them too. Bon appetite!

# BREAKFAST SUGGESTIONS

# Yogurt

Put 3-4 tablespoons of Plain, Regular yogurt in a bowl. Add a handful of blueberries, blackberries, raspberries or walnuts, pecans, shredded almonds or pine nuts. Mix well. You can also add 1-2 tablespoons of honey if you like it sweet.

# Feta Cheese

Take 2-3 tablespoons of feta cheese. Add black olives and pine nuts, walnuts or pecans. Optional: You can add mint leaves or basil leaves.

# Hard Boiled Eggs

Peel and slice two hard boiled eggs and one Avocado. You can sprinkle salt, black pepper or cayenne pepper, according to your taste.

**Tip:** You can prepare a few "hard-boiled eggs" ahead and keep them in the refrigerator for a handy, quick snack.

Caution: Use hard-boiled eggs within a few days, definitely within a week or they will spoil.

# Omelets

## Basic Omelet

Cooking Time = About 10 minutes

**Ingredients:**

Eggs = 2
Green onions = 2 (You can use 1/2 of one regular white onion in place of green onions), chopped
Olive oil = 2 tablespoons
Salt = ½ teaspoon

Add olive oil and chopped onions to a medium or large pan. Place it on stove at low heat. Cook for a few minutes until onions have softened and turned yellowish.

Meanwhile, crack open 2 eggs in a bowl. Using a tablespoon, dish out 1 egg yolk and throw it away. Leave one egg yolk. Beat it along with the egg whites. Add the eggs to the pan once onions are done.

Sprinkle the salt. In a few minutes, the eggs start looking like an omelet. With a spatula, turn the omelet over. Don't worry if it breaks down. Just turn the pieces over. Cook for a few minutes and your delicious Omelet is ready.

## Mushroom Omelet

Follow the basic omelet recipe, but use a handful of mushrooms after your onions are done. Follow the rest of the recipe.

## Spinach Omelet

Follow the basic omelet recipe. Add a handful of washed spinach leaves soon after you pour the beaten eggs in the pan. Cook another couple of minutes. Then fold it, instead of turning it over, so the spinach is all inside. Let it cool off for 2-3 minutes, before you eat.

## Bell Pepper Omelet

Follow the basic omelet recipe. Chop 1/2 of a bell pepper (any color) and add when you start with your onions. If you like spicy, you can add ½ teaspoon of Cumin seeds and ¼ to ½ teaspoon of cayenne pepper or black pepper soon after pouring the eggs.

Add a few fresh leaves of cilantro or parsley. Then fold it over, so the chopped bell pepper is all inside. Let it cool off for 2-3 minutes, before you eat.

## Avocado Omelet

Peel an avocado and slice it into chunks. Once the basic omelet is ready, add avocado chunks. Add a few fresh leaves of cilantro or parsley. Then fold it over, so the avocado chunks are all inside. Let it cool off for 2-3 minutes, before you eat.
If you like avocados, this will be a morning delight for you. Avocados help to raise your good (HDL) cholesterol and are a good source of protein.

## Spicy Omelet

Follow the basic omelet recipe. Right after you add the eggs to the pan, add ¼ to ½ teaspoon of cayenne pepper. Add ½ teaspoon of Cumin seeds. Add a few fresh leaves of cilantro or parsley. You can also use ½ of a jalapeño pepper in place of cayenne pepper.

# Healthy Crepes

Cooking Time = About 3 - 5 minutes for one crepe

Recipe makes 4 Crepes.

## Ingredients:

Mong Daal Flour = 2 tablespoons (from an Indian grocery store)
Besan = 2 tablespoons (from an Indian grocery store)
Almond flour = 2 tablespoons
Egg = 1
Himalayan Salt or Sea Salt = 1/2 teaspoon

Optional:
Cumin seeds (or powder) or Caraway seeds = 1/2 teaspoon
Black pepper or Cayenne pepper.= 1/2 teaspoon
Garlic = 1 clove, thinly sliced.


In a bowl, mix Mong daal flour, Besan and Almond flour, add small amount of water ( about 1/2 cup). Mix well. Then break one egg into the bowl. Mix well. You may need to add a little more water, till the consistency of the batter is runny.

Put a skillet on low heat. Wait a few minutes until the skillet is mildly hot. Pour about 1/4 of the batter on the skillet. Move skillet from side to side, so the batter spreads out evenly. Let it cook until it looks all dried up and edges have turned brownish and rolled-up. It takes a few minutes. With a pancake spatula, turn it over. Let it cook for another couple of minutes.

Remove crepe from skillet into a plate. Let it cool of for a minute or so. then roll it up. You can also add a filling before you roll up.

Optional:
In the beginning, add cumin (or caraway seeds), black pepper or cayenne pepper and garlic in the bowl.

---

Fillings for Crepes

Here are some ideas for the filling:

1. Cut an avocado into small pieces. Add black pepper, salt, and cayenne pepper (as optional). Add a few Cilantro leaves. Squeeze a lime or lemon.
2. Hard boiled eggs, sliced
3. Cheese
4. Salad
5. Small chicken pieces, cooked (see recipes later in the book)
6. Ground chicken/beef/turkey, cooked (see recipes later in the book)

# Scrambled Eggs - Mushrooms

Cooking Time = About 10 minutes

**Ingredients:**

Eggs = 1-2
Mushrooms = 4, diced
Green onions = 2 or a small regular onion, chopped
Garlic = 1 clove, chopped
Olive oil = 2 tablespoons
Salt = 1/2 teaspoon

Optional:

Fenugreek seeds = 1/2 teaspoon
Cumin seeds = 1/2 teaspoon
Turmeric = 1/2 teaspoon
Clove = 1/4 teaspoon
Cayenne pepper = 1/2 teaspoon OR ½ of a jalapeño, sliced
Mustard, yellow or Dijon = 1/2 teaspoon

In a pan, add olive oil, onions, garlic and salt. Start the stove at low heat and let it cook for about 5 minutes, stirring frequently. Then, add mushrooms and let it cook for another few minutes.

In a bowl, crack open 1 - 2 eggs, beat well and add to the pan. Let cook for a few minutes, stirring frequently. Cool for a couple of minutes before serving.

Optional:

In the beginning, add turmeric, fenugreek seeds, cumin seeds and clove along with the onions. At the end, you can add few cherry tomatoes, fresh cilantro or parsley leaves, fresh mint leaves or fresh basil leaves.

*Make it Spicy*: In the beginning, add ¼ to ½ teaspoon of cayenne pepper or ½ of a jalapeño pepper in place of cayenne pepper.

# Scrambled Eggs - Spinach

Cooking Time = About 10 minutes

**Ingredients:**

Eggs = 1-2
Spinach = about 1/2 cup
Green onions = 2 or a small regular onion, chopped
Garlic = 1 clove, chopped
Olive oil = 2 tablespoons
Salt = 1/2 teaspoon

Optional:

Cranberries, fresh or dried = a handful
Fenugreek seeds = 1/2 teaspoon
Cumin seeds = 1/2 teaspoon
Turmeric = 1/2 teaspoon
Clove = 1/4 teaspoon
Cayenne pepper = 1/2 teaspoon or ½ of a jalapeño pepper in place of cayenne pepper
Mustard, yellow or Dijon = 1/2 teaspoon

In a pan, add olive oil, onions, garlic and salt. Start the stove at low heat and let it cook for about 5 minutes, stirring frequently. Then add spinach and let it cook for another few minutes. In a bowl, crack open 1 - 2 eggs, beat well and add to the pan. Let cook for a few minutes, stirring frequently. Cool for a couple of minutes before serving.

Optional:

In the beginning, add a few cranberries, turmeric, fenugreek seeds, cumin seeds and clove, along with onions. At the end, you can add cherry tomatoes, fresh cilantro or parsley leaves, fresh mint leaves or fresh basil leaves.

*Make it Spicy*: In the beginning, add ¼ to ½ teaspoon of cayenne pepper OR ½ of a jalapeño pepper.

# Scrambled Eggs - Spinach - Eggplant - Bell Pepper

Cooking Time = About 15 minutes

## Ingredients:

Egg = 1-2
Spinach = about 1 cup
Eggplant = 1, preferably Japanese or Chinese, chopped
Bell pepper = 1, any color, preferably red, cut into chunks
Tomatoes = 5 cherry, halved or 1 regular, cut into chunks
Green onions = 2 or a small regular onion, chopped
Garlic = 1 clove, chopped
Mustard, yellow or Dijon = 1 tablespoon
Apple cider vinegar = 1 teaspoon
Olive oil = 2 tablespoons
Salt = 1/2 teaspoon

Optional:

Pine nuts = a handful
Fenugreek seeds = 1/2 teaspoon
Cumin seeds = 1/2 teaspoon
Turmeric = 1/2 teaspoon
Cayenne pepper = 1/2 teaspoon OR ½ of a jalapeño pepper

In a pan, add olive oil, onions, garlic and salt. Start the stove at low heat and add eggplant. Pour mustard and vinegar on eggplant chunks. Cook for about 5 minutes, stirring frequently.

In a bowl, crack open 1 - 2 eggs, beat well and add to the pan. Let cook on low heat for a few minutes, stirring frequently. Once eggs are done, add spinach, tomatoes and bell pepper. Cook for 3-5 minutes on low heat.

Optional:
In the beginning, add turmeric, fenugreek seeds and cumin seeds along with onions. In the end, add pine nuts, fresh cilantro or parsley leaves, fresh mint leaves or fresh basil leaves.

*Make it Spicy*: In the beginning, add ¼ to ½ teaspoon of cayenne pepper OR ½ of a jalapeño pepper along with onions.

# Scrambled Eggs - Broccoli - Eggplant

Cooking Time = About 15 minutes

**Ingredients:**

Egg = 1 - 2
Broccoli = about 1 cup
Eggplant = 1, preferably Japanese or Chinese, chopped
Onion = a small regular onion, chopped
Garlic = 1 clove, chopped
Olive oil = 2 tablespoons

Optional:

Pine nuts = a handful
Fenugreek seeds = 1/2 teaspoon
Cumin seeds = 1/2 teaspoon
Turmeric = 1/2 teaspoon
Cayenne pepper = 1/2 teaspoon OR ½ of a jalapeño pepper

In a pan, add one cup of water. Start the stove at low heat and add broccoli, eggplant, onions and garlic. Cover and cook for about 5 minutes, until most of the water has evaporated.

In a bowl, crack open 1 - 2 eggs, beat well and add to the pan. Let cook on low heat for a few minutes, stirring frequently. Once eggs are done, add olive oil. Cook for 1-2 minutes on low heat.

Optional:

In the beginning, add turmeric, fenugreek seeds and cumin seeds along with onions. In the end, add pine nuts, fresh cilantro or parsley leaves, fresh mint leaves or fresh basil leaves.

*Make it Spicy:* In the beginning, add ¼ to ½ teaspoon of cayenne pepper OR ½ of a jalapeño pepper along with onions.

# Scrambled Eggs - Bell Pepper - Zucchini

Cooking Time = About 15 minutes

**Ingredients:**

Eggs = 1-2
Bell pepper = 1/2 diced
Zucchini = 1/2 small, chopped
Tomato = 1, diced
Green onions = 2 or a small regular onion, chopped
Garlic = 1 clove, chopped
Olive oil = 2 tablespoons
Salt = 1/2 teaspoon

Optional:

Fig = 1, ripe
Fenugreek seeds = 1/2 teaspoon
Cumin seeds = 1/2 teaspoon
Turmeric = 1/2 teaspoon
Clove = 1/4 teaspoon
Cayenne pepper = 1/2 teaspoon OR ½ of a jalapeño, sliced
Mustard, yellow or Dijon = 1/2 teaspoon

In a pan add olive oil, zucchini, onions, garlic and salt. Start the stove at low heat and let it cook for about 5 minutes, stirring frequently. Then, add bell pepper and cook for another few minutes.

In a bowl, crack open 1 - 2 eggs, beat well and then add to the pan. Let cook for a few minutes, stirring frequently. Cool for a couple of minutes before serving.

Optional:

In the beginning, add turmeric, fenugreek seeds, cumin seeds, and clove, along with onions. At the end you can add few cherry tomatoes, fresh cilantro or parsley leaves, fresh mint leaves.

*Make it Spicy*: In the beginning, add ¼ to ½ teaspoon of cayenne pepper OR ½ of a jalapeño pepper and add about 1/2 teaspoon of yellow mustard.

*Make it Sweet*: At the end, add one ripe fig and fresh basil leaves.

# Scrambled Eggs - Bell Pepper - Cauliflower

Cooking Time = About 20 minutes

**Ingredients:**

Eggs = 1-2
Bell pepper = 1/2 of regular sized bell pepper, any color. Cut into several pieces
Cauliflower = 1/8 of the whole cauliflower head, chopped into 4-6 small pieces
Onion = 1/2 of a medium sized onion, chopped
Garlic = 1 clove, sliced
Olive oil = 3 tablespoons
Vinegar = 1/2 teaspoon
Lemon, fresh = Cut in half
Dijon Mustard (or regular, yellow) = small amount
Salt = 1/2 teaspoon

Optional:

Pine nuts = a handful
Cumin seeds (or powder) or Caraway seeds = 1/2 teaspoon
Turmeric powder = 1/2 teaspoon
Clove powder = 1/4 teaspoon
Black pepper OR Cayenne pepper = 1/2 teaspoon
Cilantro or Basil or Mint leaves = 8 -10


In a regular frying pan, pour 1 cup of water. Add mustard and salt. Squeeze the juice of 1/2 lemon. Stir.  Place it on the stove at <u>medium</u> heat. Add cauliflower and cover it. Let it cook for about <u>10</u> minutes. Check only once or twice to make sure the water has not cooked off. Avoid frequent uncovering. It will reduce the amount of steam, which is cooking the cauliflower.

Uncover, lower the heat. Add olive oil, onion, and garlic.

Stir frequently. DO NOT COVER. In about 3-5 minutes, when there is very little water left, add one or two beaten eggs.

Scramble it with the spatula. Let it cook for about 3-5 minutes, until eggs are done. Stir frequently.

Add bell pepper and cook for another 3-5 minutes. In the end, add vinegar, a handful of pine nuts and cilantro, basil or mint leaves. Mix well.

Optional: In the beginning, add clove powder, turmeric powder, cumin (or caraway seeds), black pepper OR cayenne pepper.

# Scrambled Eggs - Mushroom - Okra - Lentils

Cooking Time = About 20 minutes

**Ingredients:**

Eggs = 1 - 2
Mushrooms, Shiitake = 2, each cut into medium pieces.
Okra = 8-10, each sliced into 2 - 3 piece
Lentils = 2 tablespoons. (You can get it from an India/Pakistani grocery store.)
Onion = 1/2 of a medium sized onion, chopped
Garlic = 1 clove, sliced
Olive oil = 3 tablespoons
Olives = Black, pitted; 6-8, cut into small pieces.
Vinegar, Balsamic = 1/2 teaspoon
Lemon, fresh = Cut in half
Salt = 1/2 teaspoon
Cumin seeds (or powder) or Caraway seeds = 1/2 teaspoon
Turmeric powder = 1/2 teaspoon
Basil leaves = 8 -10 fresh or 1 tablespoon of dried leaves

Optional:
Black pepper OR Cayenne pepper = 1/2 teaspoon
Clove powder = 1/4 teaspoon

    In a regular frying pan, add two tablespoons of olive oil, onion, and garlic. Cook at low heat until onions turn yellowish and soft, which takes about 5 minutes.

    Pour 1 cup of water into pan. Add cumin seeds, turmeric, and salt. Squeeze and add the juice of 1/2 lemon.

    Add okra and lentils. Stir and cover it. Let it cook for about 10 minutes on low heat. Check only once or twice to make sure the water has not cooked off. Avoid frequent uncovering. It will reduce the amount of steam, which is cooking the okra and lentils.

Add one or two beaten eggs. Scramble with the spatula. Let it cook for about 3-5 minutes, until eggs are done. Stir frequently.

Add mushrooms, olives and basil leaves. Add one tablespoon of olive oil and 1/2 teaspoon of Balsamic vinegar. Mix well. Cook for another 1-2 minutes.

Optional: In the beginning, add clove powder, black pepper OR cayenne pepper.

# Scrambled Eggs - Bell Pepper - Green Beans

Cooking Time = About 15 minutes

**Ingredients:**

Eggs = 1 - 2
Bell pepper = 1 diced
Green Beans = 10
Tomato = 1, diced
Green onions = 2 or a small, regular onion, chopped
Garlic = 1 clove, chopped
Olive oil = 2 tablespoons
White Vinegar = 1/2 teaspoon

Optional:

Cranberries, fresh or dried = a handful
Fenugreek seeds = 1/2 teaspoon
Cumin seeds = 1/2 teaspoon
Turmeric = 1/2 teaspoon
Cayenne pepper = 1/2 teaspoon OR ½ of a jalapeño

In a pan, add a small amount of water and olive oil. Add green beans, onions and garlic. Start the stove at medium heat and let cook for about 5 minutes, stirring frequently. Do not cover. Then, add tomatoes, bell pepper and white vinegar. Let cook for another few minutes.

In a bowl, crack open 1 - 2 eggs, beat well and add to the pan. Let cook for a few minutes, stirring frequently. Cool for a couple of minutes before serving.

Optional:

In the beginning, add cranberries, turmeric, fenugreek seeds and cumin seeds along with onions. At the end, you can add fresh oregano or thyme leaves.

*Make it Spicy*: In the beginning, add ¼ to ½ teaspoon of cayenne pepper OR ½ of a jalapeño pepper.

# Scrambled Eggs - Eggplant- Green Beans

Cooking Time = About 15 minutes

**Ingredients:**

Egg = 1
Green Beans = 10
Eggplant = one, sliced.
Onion = a small, regular onion, chopped
Garlic = 1 clove, chopped
Olives, black, pitted = 6, sliced
Olive oil = 1 tablespoon
Basil leaves = 6 fresh or 1 teaspoon of dried leaves

Optional:

Fenugreek seeds = 1/2 teaspoon
Cumin seeds = 1/2 teaspoon
Turmeric = 1/2 teaspoon
Cayenne pepper = 1/2 teaspoon powder OR ½ of a fresh cayenne pepper or jalapeño pepper


In a pan, add 1/2 cup of water and olive oil.  Add eggplant, green beans, onions and garlic. Start the stove at low heat, cover and let cook for about 5 minutes, stirring frequently.

In a bowl, crack open 1 egg, beat well and add to the pan. Let cook for a few minutes, uncovered, stirring frequently. Add basil leaves and sliced olives. Cool for a couple of minutes before serving.

Optional:

In the beginning, add turmeric, fenugreek seeds and cumin seeds along with onions.
*Make it Spicy*: In the beginning, add ¼ to ½ teaspoon of cayenne pepper powder OR ½ of a fresh jalapeño or cayenne pepper, cut into small pieces.

# Zesty Scrambled Eggs - Green Beans - Eggplant

Cooking Time = About 20 minutes

**Ingredients:**

Eggs = 1-2
Green beans = 15
Eggplant = 1/2, preferably Japanese or Chinese.
Cinnamon stick = 1
Tomato = 1, medium size
Yogurt = Plain, 2-3 tablespoons
Garlic = 1 clove, sliced
Olive oil = 3 tablespoons
Lemon, fresh = Cut into two halves
Dijon Mustard (or regular, yellow) = small amount
Salt = 1/2 teaspoon

Optional:

Pine nuts = a handful
Bay leaf = 1
Cumin seeds (or powder) or Caraway seeds = 1/2 teaspoon
Turmeric powder = 1/2 teaspoon
Cloves powder = 1/4 teaspoon
Black pepper OR Cayenne pepper = 1/2 teaspoon
Cilantro or Basil or Mint leaves = 8-10


In a regular frying pan, pour 1/2 cup of water. Add mustard and salt. Squeeze 1/2 lemon. Stir and cook at <u>medium</u> heat. Add green beans, eggplant, cinnamon stick and bay leaf. DO NOT COVER. Let cook for about <u>5</u> minutes. Stir occasionally. Lower the heat. Add olive oil, garlic, yogurt and tomato.

Stir frequently. DO NOT COVER. In about <u>10</u> minutes, add one or two beaten eggs. Scramble it with a spatula. Let it cook for another 3 - 5 minutes, until eggs are done. Stir frequently. In the end, add a handful of pine nuts and cilantro leaves (or basil or mint leaves).

<u>Optional</u>:

In the beginning, add bay leaf, clove powder, turmeric powder, cumin (or caraway seeds), powdered black pepper (or powdered cayenne pepper).

# Scrambled Eggs - Bell Pepper - Zucchini - Daikon Radish

Cooking Time = About 15 minutes

**Ingredients:**

Eggs = 1-2
Bell pepper = 1/2, diced
Zucchini = 1/2, sliced
Daikon Radish = 4 inch piece, peeled and cut in small pieces
Green onions = 2 or a small regular onion, chopped
Garlic = 1 clove, chopped
Olive oil = 2 tablespoons
Salt = 1/2 teaspoon

Optional:

Pine nuts = a handful
Fenugreek seeds = 1/2 teaspoon
Cumin seeds = 1/2 teaspoon
Turmeric = 1/2 teaspoon
Clove = 1/4 teaspoon
Cayenne pepper = 1/2 teaspoon OR ½ of a jalapeño, sliced
Mustard, yellow or Dijon = 1/2 teaspoon
Cherry tomatoes = 5-8
Fresh cilantro, mint or basil leaves = 8-10
Figs = 2 ripe

    In a frying pan, add olive oil, zucchini, Daikon radish and onions. Place the pan on stove at low heat.

Optional: Add garlic, turmeric, fenugreek seeds, cumin seeds, and clove.

    Sprinkle salt. Let cook for about 5 minutes, stirring frequently. Then, add bell pepper and let cook for another few minutes.

In a bowl, beat 1 - 2 eggs and then add to the pan. Let it cook for a few minutes, stirring frequently. Let it cool for a couple of minutes before serving.

Optional:

At the end, add a few cherry tomatoes, pine nuts, fresh cilantro, mint or basil leaves.

*Make it Spicy*: In the beginning, add cayenne pepper OR jalapeño pepper and add mustard.

*Make it Sweet*: Add two ripe figs, chopped and a few fresh basil leaves.

# Scrambled Eggs - Pumpkin

Cooking Time = About 15 minutes

**Ingredients:**

Eggs = 1 - 2
Pumpkin, fresh = 10 small slices, about 1/4 inch thick, 2 inches wide and 2 inches long, peeled.
Celery Stick = 1, cut into small pieces
Olive oil = 2 tablespoons
Vinegar = 1/2 teaspoon
Lemon, fresh = Cut in half
Mustard, regular, yellow = small amount
Salt = 1 teaspoon
Cumin seeds (or powder) or Caraway seeds = 1 teaspoon
Garlic = 1 clove, sliced

Optional:

Black Pepper OR Cayenne pepper = 1/2 teaspoon.


A wok works better, but you can use a regular frying pan. Add olive oil, pumpkin and celery slices to the wok. Place it on the stove at medium heat. Stir frequently. DO NOT COVER. In about 10 minutes, pumpkin slices will be done: softened but not mushy.

Turn the heat down to low. Add the mustard and squeeze the juice of 1/2 lemon directly on the pumpkin slices. Add vinegar, garlic, cumin seeds, and salt. Let it cook another 2-3 minutes, stirring frequently.

Add beaten eggs to the wok. After a minute, scramble it. Cook for another 2 - 3 minutes.

Optional:

Make it Hot: In the beginning, add Cayenne OR Black Pepper on the pumpkin slices.

# Scrambled Eggs - Green Beans - Bell Pepper - Tomatoes - Turnip

Cooking Time = About 15 minutes

**Ingredients:**

Eggs = 1-2
Green beans = 4-6
Bell pepper = 1/2, diced
Tomatoes = 1-2, diced
Turnip = 1/2, peeled and diced
Green onions = 2 or a small regular onion, chopped
Garlic = 1 clove, chopped
Olive oil = 2 tablespoons
Salt = 1/2 teaspoon
Lemon = Cut in half.

Optional:

Fenugreek seeds = 1/2 teaspoon
Cumin seeds = 1/2 teaspoon
Turmeric = 1/2 teaspoon
Cayenne pepper = 1/2 teaspoon OR ½ of a jalapeño, sliced
Mustard, yellow or Dijon = 1/2 teaspoon
Fresh cilantro leaves = 8-10

In a frying pan, add olive oil, 1/2 cup of water, turnip, onion, garlic, and salt. Squeeze lemon directly onto the pan.

Optional: Add fenugreek seeds, cumin seeds, turmeric, cayenne pepper and mustard.

Cover and cook on low heat for about 10 minutes, stirring occasionally to make sure water is still there. Then, add bell pepper, green beans, and tomatoes. Let it cook for another few minutes, uncovered. Add beaten eggs to the pan. After a minute, scramble it Cook for another 2 - 3 minutes. In the end, add cilantro leaves.

# LUNCH OR DINNER

*You can use any of the scrambled eggs recipes for lunch or dinner.*

# VEGETABLE DISHES

# Lettuce Wraps: Cheese - Avocado - Eggs

**Ingredients:**

Lettuce = 1 head of Iceberg lettuce
Cheese, feta or cottage = a small amount
Avocado = 1, peeled, sliced
Eggs= 2, boiled, peeled, sliced
Almonds, sliced = 2 tablespoon
Salt = a tiny amount

Gently peel off a leaf from the lettuce head. Place the cheese, avocado slices and egg slices in the center of the lettuce leaf. Top it with sliced almonds. Sprinkle a tiny amount of salt. Roll up the lettuce leaf into a wrap. You can make about 4 wraps with this recipe.

# SALADS

## Cucumber - Tomato - Yogurt Salad

**Ingredients:**

Yogurt, plain = 4 tablespoons
Tomatoes, cherry = 6 - 10
Cucumber = 1 medium sized, cut into pieces
Green Onion = 1 sliced. Also use green portion
Salt = 1/2 teaspoon
Cumin seeds = 1/2 teaspoon
Mint leaves or basil leaves (preferably fresh) = a few

Add yogurt to a medium sized bowl. Dilute it by adding and mixing 2 tablespoons of water. Then, add onion, cucumber, cumin seeds, salt and mix well. Then mix in tomatoes and mint leaves. Your salad is ready.

## Cucumber - Tomato - Avocado - Walnut Salad

**Ingredients:**
Lettuce = a few leaves, chopped
Cucumber = 1/2, sliced
Tomato = 1 medium, cut into large pieces OR about 10 cherry tomatoes, whole
Avocado = 1, peeled, sliced
Onion = preferably red, 1/2, peeled, cut into slices
Walnuts, shelled = a handful
Balsamic Vinegar = a tiny amount
Lime or Lemon = 1, cut in half
Salt = a tiny amount

In a medium size bowl, add chopped lettuce. Then, add chopped onion, tomatoes and avocado. Mix well. Add walnuts. Sprinkle salt and a tiny amount of Balsamic Vinegar. In the end, squeeze lime. Mix well.

# Olive - Pine Nut - Avocado Salad

## Ingredients:

Olives, black or green = 8-10
Pine nuts = a handful
Avocado = 1, peeled, sliced
Lettuce = a few leaves, chopped
Tomato = 1 medium, cut into large pieces OR about 10 cherry tomatoes, whole
Balsamic Vinegar = a tiny amount
Lime or Lemon = 1, cut in half
Salt = a tiny amount.

In a bowl, add chopped lettuce. Squeeze lemon juice and sprinkle salt and a tiny amount of Balsamic Vinegar. Then add pine nuts, olives, tomatoes and avocado. Mix well.

# Papaya - Spinach - Almond Salad

## Ingredients:

Lettuce, Romaine = half cup, chopped
Arugula = half cup, chopped
Spinach, baby = half cup
Cucumber = 1/2, sliced
Papaya = 1, small, peeled, seeds removed and cut into chunks
Tomato = 1, medium, cut into large pieces OR about 10 cherry tomatoes, whole
Almonds, sliced = two tablespoons
Balsamic Vinegar = a tiny amount
Lime or Lemon = 1, cut in half

In a bowl, add baby spinach, chopped lettuce and arugula. Squeeze lemon juice and add a tiny amount of Balsamic Vinegar. Then add cucumber, sliced almonds and tomatoes. In the end, add papaya. Mix gently.

# Pesto

## Ingredients

Basil leaves, fresh = 1 cup
Spinach, baby = 1/2 cup
Parsley/Cilantro leaves, fresh = 1/4 cup
Lemon = 3, cut into half
Onions, red = 1/2, cut into small pieces
Garlic = 2 cloves, cut into small pieces
Cheese, parmesan = 1/2 cup
Salt, Himalayan = 1 teaspoon
Olive oil = 2-3 tablespoons


Put all of the ingredients, except lemon, in a Food Processor. Then squeeze lemon halves. Grind for a couple of minutes, until, a thick paste is formed.

Optional: Add a handful of pine nuts.


Note: You can use pesto as a salad dressing. Additionally, put a tablespoon into any of the recipes in this book. Try and taste. Be adventurous!

# Spaghetti Squash  Recipes

Spaghetti squash is a great substitute for pasta, rice and quinoa, especially for diabetics. The problem is that most people don't know how to cook it. In addition, there is even bigger problem: It has a bland taste.

In this section, you will learn how to overcome both of these problems. Then, you will have easy to cook, delicious, healthy spaghetti squash dishes.

## How to Cook Spaghetti Squash

First get your oven going: Bake at 375 F. In the meantime, cut the spaghetti squash lengthwise into two halves. Scrap and remove the seeds and pulp.

Place both pieces in the heated oven, rind side up. Bake for about 40 - 45 minutes.

Remove from the spaghetti squash halves from the oven, using oven mitts, as it gets very hot. Let it cool of for about 5 minutes. Then, take one piece at a time and put it in a plate. Run a fork through the flesh, lengthwise. Flesh will come up in strands, like spaghetti, hence the name spaghetti squash.

## How To Make Spaghetti Squash Tasty

There are several ways you can make spaghetti squash taste zesty.

1. Squeeze the juice of a lemon over the spaghetti squash. Add a small amount of Himalayan or Sea salt, and vinegar, Balsamic or Apple-cider, to the spaghetti squash and mix well. Garnish with a few fresh Mint or Basil leaves. You can also add a handful of pine nuts, sliced almonds or walnuts.

2. Add red onions, chopped into small pieces, a few capers, black olives, cherry tomatoes and fresh Mint leaves to the spaghetti squash. Add a small amount of Himalayan or Sea salt, and vinegar, Balsamic or Apple-cider, to the spaghetti squash and mix

well. You can also add a handful of pine nuts, sliced almonds or walnuts.

3. Prepare the following sauce and put it on the spaghetti squash. Mix well.

In a small pot, add two tablespoons of Lentils (whole, with skin), 1/2 cup of water, a small amount of salt, turmeric, caraway seeds, black (or red) pepper and coriander powder. Add 1/2 onion, chopped, and one clove of garlic, chopped.
Let it cook at low heat for about 30 minutes, covered, until Lentils have softened and no water is left. Add 1 tablespoon of olive oil. Garnish with a few fresh Mint or Basil leaves.

4. Add any of the scrambled eggs or meat dishes from this book, to the spaghetti squash. Mix well.

# Pumpkin Z-Fries

Cooking Time = About 15 minutes

**Ingredients:**

Pumpkin, fresh = Cut into the size of French Fries, about 20 - 25,
some peeled and some unpeeled
Olive oil = 2 tablespoons
Cheddar cheese, shredded = a handful
Mustard, Dijon = 3 teaspoons
Vinegar = 1/2 teaspoon

Optional:

Garlic powder = 1 teaspoon
Salt = 1/2 teaspoon
Cumin seeds (or powder) or Caraway seeds = 1 teaspoon
Black Pepper = 1 teaspoon OR Cayenne pepper = 1/2 teaspoon


Place a frying pan on medium heat. Warm olive oil and
then, add pumpkin fries. Add Dijon mustard directly on the
pumpkin fries.

Optional: Add vinegar, garlic, cumin seeds, salt and black OR
cayenne pepper.

Cook for about 10 minutes. DO NOT COVER. Turn the
pumpkin fries over a few times, so they don't get burned.

Turn the heat down to low. Sprinkle a handful of shredded
cheddar cheese. It will melt in a couple of minutes. Place
Pumpkin Z-Fries on paper towel to soak up excess oil.

# Pumpkin Z-Fries - Scrambled Eggs - Eggplant

Cooking Time = About 15 minutes

## Ingredients:

Eggs = 2
Pumpkin, fresh = Cut into the size of French Fries, about 20 - 25, some peeled and some unpeeled
Eggplant = 1 Japanese or Chinese or 2 small round ones; sliced
Olive oil = 3 tablespoons
Cheddar cheese, shredded = a handful
Mustard, Dijon = 3 teaspoons
Vinegar = 1/2 teaspoon

Optional:
Garlic powder = 1 teaspoon
Salt = 1/2 teaspoon
Cumin seeds (or powder) or Caraway seeds = 1 teaspoon
Onion, Green = 2, chopped. (You can use a small regular onion instead)
Black Pepper = 1 teaspoon OR Cayenne pepper = 1/2 teaspoon
Fresh or dried thyme, oregano, mint OR basil leaves

In a pan, add olive oil, pumpkin fries, and eggplant slices. Add mustard directly on the pumpkin fries.

Optional: Add vinegar, garlic, cumin seeds, salt and black or cayenne pepper.

Cook for about 10 minutes on <u>medium</u> heat. DO NOT COVER. Turn the pumpkin fries and eggplant slices over a few times, so they don't get burned. Then, turn the heat down to low. Sprinkle in a handful of shredded cheddar cheese. In a few minutes, add onions and beaten eggs to the pan. Let it cook about 1 minute, then scramble the eggs with a spatula. Cook for another 2 - 3 minutes, stirring frequently. In the end, add fresh or dried oregano, thyme, mint or basil leaves.

# Zucchini Z-Fries - Avocado

Cooking Time = About 15 minutes

**Ingredients:**

Zucchini, fresh = Unpeeled, cut into the size of French Fries, about 20-25
Avocado = 1, peeled, sliced
Cherry tomatoes = about 10
Olive oil = 3 tablespoons
Cheddar cheese, shredded = a handful
Mustard, Dijon = 4-5 teaspoons
Garlic powder = 1 teaspoon
Onion, Green = 2, chopped (You can use a small regular onion instead.)

Optional:

Salt = 1/2 teaspoon
Clove powder = 1/2 teaspoon
Cumin seeds (or powder) or Caraway seeds = 1 teaspoon
Black Pepper = 1 teaspoon OR Cayenne pepper = 1/2 teaspoon
Cilantro leaves = 8-10 fresh or dried = 1 teaspoon


In a regular frying pan, add olive oil and zucchini fries . Sprinkle garlic powder and add mustard directly on the zucchini fries.

Optional : Add clove powder, cumin seeds, salt and black or cayenne pepper directly on the zucchini fries.

Cook for about 5 minutes on medium heat. DO NOT COVER. Turn the zucchini fries over a few times, so they don't get burned. Sprinkle a handful of shredded cheddar cheese directly on the zucchini fries. Once the cheese melts, remove the zucchini fries onto a plate. Top it with chopped onions, cherry tomatoes, avocado slices and cilantro leaves.

# Pumpkin Stir Fry

Cooking Time = About 15 minutes

**Ingredients:**

Pumpkin, fresh = 10 small slices, about 1/4 inch thick, 2 inches wide and 2 inches long, peeled
Celery Stick = 1, cut into small pieces
Olive oil = 2 tablespoons
Vinegar = 1/2 teaspoon
Lemon, fresh = Cut in half.
Mustard, regular, yellow = small amount
Salt = 1 teaspoon
Cumin seeds (or powder) or Caraway seeds = 1 teaspoon
Garlic = 1 clove, sliced
Black Pepper = 1 teaspoon OR Cayenne pepper = 1/2 teaspoon

Optional:
Avocado slices
Mint or Basil leaves = 8-10


A wok works better, but you can use a regular frying pan. Warm olive oil on <u>medium</u> heat. Add pumpkin slices and celery slices. Stir frequently. DO NOT COVER. In about 10 minutes, pumpkin slices will be done: softened but not mushy.

Turn the heat down to low. Add mustard and 1/2 lemon juice directly on the pumpkin slices. Add vinegar, garlic, cumin seeds, salt and cayenne pepper (or black pepper) to the wok. Let it cook another 2-3 minutes, stirring frequently.

Optional:
For variety, add Avocado slices at the end. Let it cook another 2-3 minutes, stirring frequently. In the end, add a few Mint or Basil leaves.

# Zucchini - Eggplant - Avocado Delight

Cooking Time = About 15 minutes

## Ingredients:

Zucchini = 1 medium size, unpeeled, sliced
Eggplant = 1 small, preferably Japanese or Chinese, sliced
Avocado = 1, peeled, sliced into chunks
Yogurt = Plain, 2 tablespoons
Tomato = 1 medium size, sliced
Onion = 1/2 of a medium sized onion
Olive oil = 3 tablespoons

Optional:

Walnuts or pecans = a handful
Clove, powder = a pinch
Garlic = 1 clove, sliced
Cumin seeds (or powder) or Caraway seeds = 1/2 teaspoon
Turmeric powder = 1/2 teaspoon
Black pepper OR Cayenne pepper = 1/2 teaspoon
Oregano, thyme or rosemary leaves = about 1 teaspoon

In a regular frying pan on medium heat, add olive oil and chopped onions. Stir frequently. In about 3-5 minutes, onion will turn yellowish.

Lower the heat. Add sliced Zucchini and eggplant. After about 2-3 minutes, add yogurt. Let it cook for about 10 minutes on low heat. DO NOT COVER. Stir frequently.

Add Avocado slices and tomato slices. Cook for another couple of minutes. In the end, add walnuts and oregano or thyme or rosemary leaves.

Optional: In the beginning, add clove powder, turmeric powder, cumin (or caraway seeds), black pepper, cayenne pepper.

# Zucchini - Bell Pepper - Green Beans - Mushrooms

Cooking Time = About 15 minutes

**Ingredients:**

Zucchini = 1, small, unpeeled, sliced
Bell pepper, red = 1, cut into pieces
Green beans = small, 8-10
Mushrooms = white, 5, cut into halves
Tomato = 1 medium, sliced
Onion = 1 small, chopped
Olive oil = 1 tablespoon
Mustard - yellow or Dijon = a small amount
Vinegar, Balsamic = a small amount

Optional:

Cumin seeds (or powder) or Caraway seeds = 1/2 teaspoon.
Turmeric powder = 1/2 teaspoon.
Black pepper OR Cayenne pepper = 1/2 teaspoon.
Basil or Oregano leaves =  8-10


In a regular frying pan, add 1/2 cup of water, olive oil, onion and mustard. Put on low heat, cover and stir only a couple of times. In about 5 minutes, uncover and add green beans, zucchini and tomatoes. Cook for about 5 minutes on medium heat. DO NOT COVER. Stir frequently.

Then, add bell pepper and mushrooms. Cook for about 2-3 minutes. In the end, add basil leaves or thyme leave and sprinkle with a small amount of vinegar.

Optional:
In the beginning, add cumin (or caraway seeds), black pepper OR cayenne pepper.

# Cauliflower - Pumpkin - Turnip Stir Fry

Cooking Time = About 15 minutes

## Ingredients:

Pumpkin, fresh = 15 small slices,  about 1/4 inch thick, 2 inches wide and 2 inches long, peeled
Cauliflower = 3 - 5 florets
Turnip = 1/2, peeled and cut into small slices
Celery Stick = 1, cut into small slices
Olive oil = 2 tablespoons
Vinegar = 1/2 teaspoon
Lemon, fresh = Cut in half
Mustard, regular, yellow = small amount
Salt = 1 teaspoon
Cumin seeds (or powder) or Caraway seeds = 1 teaspoon
Garlic = 1 clove, sliced
Mint leaves Or Basil leaves, fresh = 8-10 OR dried = 1 teaspoon

Optional
Black Pepper = 1 teaspoon OR Cayenne pepper = 1/2 teaspoon


A wok works better, but you can use a regular frying pan instead. Place the wok on <u>medium</u> heat. Add olive oil, pumpkin slices, turnip slices, cauliflower florets and celery slices to the wok. Stir frequently. DO NOT COVER. In about 10 minutes, pumpkin slices will be done: softened but not mushy.

Turn the heat down to low. Add mustard and 1/2 lemon juice directly on the pumpkin slices. Add vinegar, garlic, cumin seeds and salt.

<u>Optional:</u> Add cayenne pepper OR black pepper to the wok.

Let it cook another 2-3 minutes, stirring frequently

# Eggplant - Bell Pepper - Daikon Radish

Cooking Time = About 15 minutes

**Ingredients:**

Eggplant = 1 small, preferably Japanese or Chinese, sliced
Bell pepper = 1/2, cut into pieces
Daikon radish = about a 4 inch piece, peeled and cut into pieces
Yogurt = Plain, 2 tablespoons
Tomato = 1 medium size, sliced
Olive oil = 3 tablespoons
Mustard - yellow or Dijon = a small amount

Optional:

Cumin seeds (or powder) or Caraway seeds = 1/2 teaspoon
Turmeric powder = 1/2 teaspoon
Black pepper OR Cayenne pepper = 1/2 teaspoon
Basil or thyme leaves =  8-10


In a regular frying pan, add 1/2 cup of water, olive oil, eggplant and Daikon radish. Put on low heat, cover and stir only a couple of times. In about 5 minutes, uncover and add yogurt and tomato.

Optional: Add cumin (or caraway seeds), black pepper OR cayenne pepper.

Cook for about 5 minutes on low heat. DO NOT COVER. Stir frequently.

Add bell pepper and cook for about 2-3 minutes. Add a small amount of mustard and cook for another 2-3 minutes.  In the end, add basil leaves or thyme leaves.

# Cauliflower, Bell Pepper, Green Beans, Cherry Tomatoes and Green Grapes

Cooking Time = About 15 minutes

## Ingredients:

Cauliflower = 1/8 of the whole cauliflower head, chopped into 4-6 small pieces
Bell pepper = 1/2 of regular sized bell pepper, any color. Cut into 4-5 chunks
Eggplant = 1/2 of a Chinese or Japanese eggplant, cut into chunks
Green grapes = about 20
Green Beans, small = 5-10
Cherry Tomatoes = 5-10
Onion = 1/2 of a regular sized onion
Garlic = 1 clove, sliced
Olive oil = 3 tablespoons
Mustard, Dijon, (or regular, yellow) = small amount
Salt = 1/2 teaspoon
Pine nuts = a handful
Cilantro or basil leaves = 1/2 teaspoon

Optional:
Cumin seeds (or powder) or Caraway seeds = 1/2 teaspoon
Turmeric powder = 1/2 teaspoon
Black pepper OR Cayenne pepper = 1/2 teaspoon.


In a regular frying pan on low heat, add olive oil and 1/2 cup of water. Add mustard, salt, cauliflower and eggplant, and cover. Let it cook for about 10 minutes. Check only once or twice to make sure water is still in there. Uncover and raise the heat to medium. Add onion, garlic, cherry tomatoes, green beans and grapes. Stir frequently. DO NOT COVER. Add a handful of pine nuts, and basil OR cilantro leaves.

Optional: In the beginning, add cumin (or caraway seeds), turmeric, black pepper OR cayenne pepper.

---

# Nopal (Cactus) - Eggplant - Lentils

Cooking Time = About 15 minutes

## Ingredients:

Nopal = Cut in small pieces, about 1/2 cup. You can get it from a Mexican grocery store.
Eggplant = 1 small, preferably Japanese or Chinese, sliced
Lentils (with skin), also called Masoor in an Indian-Pakistani grocery store = 2 tablespoon
Garlic = 1 clove, sliced
Cumin seeds (or powder) or Caraway seeds = 1/2 teaspoon
Turmeric powder = 1/2 teaspoon
Black pepper OR Cayenne pepper = 1/2 teaspoon
Salt = 1/2 teaspoon
Onion, red = 1/4 of a medium sized onion, chopped into small pieces.
Olive oil = 2 tablespoons
Vinegar = Balsamic or Apple cider, 1 teaspoon
Lime or lemon = 1, sliced into 2
Sliced almonds or Pine nuts = a handful
Basil or Mint leaves, fresh = a few. Alternatively, use 1 teaspoon of dried leaves.

In a regular frying pan on low heat, add 1/2 cup of water, nopal, eggplant, lentils and all of the spices: garlic, cumin turmeric, black (or red) pepper and salt. Let it cook for about 10 minutes, covered, until lentils get softened and no water is left. Stir occasionally.

Uncover. Add olive oil, vinegar, onions, sliced almonds (or pine nuts) and basil (or mint) leaves to the pan. Squeeze lime (or lemon) on top of the dish. Mix well.

# Bitter Melon - Eggplant - Chana Daal - Eggs

Cooking Time = About 20 minutes

## Ingredients:

Bitter Melon = 1/4 of one bitter melon, sliced. You can get it from Indian-Pakistani-Asian grocery store.
Chana Daal = 2 tablespoon, You can get it from Indian-Pakistani grocery store
Eggplant = 1 small, preferably Japanese or Chinese, sliced
Eggs = two
Garlic = 1 clove, sliced
Cumin seeds (or powder) or Caraway seeds = 1/2 teaspoon
Turmeric powder = 1/2 teaspoon
Black pepper OR Cayenne pepper = 1/2 teaspoon
Salt = 1/2 teaspoon
Onion, red = 1/4 of a medium sized onion, chopped into small pieces.
Olive oil = 2 tablespoons
Vinegar = Balsamic or Apple cider, 1 teaspoon
Lime or lemon = 1, sliced into 2
Sliced almonds or Pine nuts = a handful
Mint or Basil leaves, fresh = a few. Alternatively, use 1 teaspoon of dried leaves.

In a regular frying pan on low heat, add 1 cup of water, bitter melon, eggplant, Chana Daal and all of the spices: garlic, cumin turmeric, black (or red) pepper and salt. Let it cook for about 15 minutes, covered, until Chana Daal get softened and no water is left. Stir occasionally.

Uncover. Add beat-up eggs, olive oil, onions, sliced almonds (or pine nuts) and mint (or basil) leaves to the pan. Let it cook for another 2 - 3 minutes, until eggs are cooked. Stir well. Add vinegar and squeeze lime (or lemon) on top of the dish. Mix well.

# Bitter Melon - Chana Daal - Spinach - Bell pepper

Cooking Time = About 20 minutes

## Ingredients:

Bitter melon = 1/4 of one bitter melon, sliced. You can get it from Indian-Pakistani-Asian grocery store.
Chana Daal = 2 tablespoon, You can get it from Indian-Pakistani grocery store
Spinach = A handful, chopped
Bell Pepper = One, preferably red, chopped
Garlic = 1 clove, sliced
Cumin seeds (or powder) or Caraway seeds = 1/2 teaspoon
Turmeric powder = 1/2 teaspoon
Black pepper OR Cayenne pepper = 1/2 teaspoon
Salt = 1/2 teaspoon
Onion, red = 1/4 of a medium sized onion, chopped into small pieces.
Olive oil = 2 tablespoons
Sliced almonds or walnuts= a handful
Mint or Basil leaves, fresh =  a few. Alternatively, use 1 teaspoon of dried leaves.
Pesto ( from recipe on page 315), 1 tablespoon

In a regular frying pan on low heat, add 1 cup of water, bitter melon, Chana Daal and all of the spices: garlic, cumin turmeric, black (or red) pepper and salt. Let it cook for about 15 minutes, covered, until Chana Daal get softened and no water is left. Stir occasionally.

Uncover. Add spinach, bell pepper, olive oil, onions, sliced almonds (or walnuts) and mint (or basil) leaves to the pan. Let it cook for another 2 - 3 minutes. Stir well. Add pesto on top of the dish. Mix well.

# 5-Leaf Saag

Cooking time = about 60 minutes

**Ingredients:**

Spinach, baby = 4 cups, chopped
Mustard greens = 6 cups, chopped
Daikon Radish Leaves = 3 cups, chopped
Arugula = 1 cup, chopped
Turnip Leaves = 1 cup, chopped
Daikon Radish = 1, peeled, chopped
Olive oil = 10 tablespoons
Butter = 1 stick
Onion = 2 medium, chopped
Garlic = 2 cloves, sliced
Vinegar = Any type, preferably Balsamic, 1 teaspoon
Salt = 1 teaspoon
Turmeric powder = 1/2 teaspoon
Cilantro leaves = a few
Lime or lemon = 1, cut in half

Optional:

Cumin seeds = 1 teaspoon
Clove powder = 1/2 teaspoon
Black pepper= 2 teaspoons OR Cayenne pepper = 1 teaspoon


In a large pot, add olive oil. Then add two chopped onions, garlic and salt. Cook on low heat for about 5 minutes, stirring frequently, until the onions have turned yellowish brown.

Add spinach, mustard greens, Daikon radish and Daikon radish leaves, turnip leaves, arugula, turmeric powder, salt and vinegar.

Cook for about 45 minutes at low heat, uncovered, stirring frequently until it is not runny and has thick consistency.

Then, pour it into a blender and grind on low until all leaves are well ground. Pour it back into the large pot.

Add 1 stick of butter. Cook for another 15 - 20 minutes on low heat, uncovered, until you start to see oil separating at the periphery.

In the end, add cilantro. Squeeze and add lime or lemon. Mix well. Let it sit for about 15 minutes before serving.

Optional:
In the beginning, add black pepper OR cayenne pepper and clove powder and cumin seeds.

# MEAT/POULTRY DISHES

# Chicken Nuggets
(Kids and teenagers love them)

Cooking Time = About 30 - 45 minutes

## Ingredients:

Chicken = Boneless, preferably breast, about 1 Lb., cut into pieces about 2 x 1 inches
Yogurt = 3 tablespoons
Olive oil = 2 tablespoon
Lime or lemon = 1, cut in half
Apple cider vinegar = 1 teaspoon
Mustard, Dijon = 1 teaspoon
Garlic powder = 1 tablespoon
Sea-Salt = 1 teaspoon

Optional:

Cayenne pepper or black pepper = 1/2 teaspoon


In a large pan, add olive oil, yogurt, apple cider vinegar, Dijon mustard, garlic powder and salt. Squeeze lime or lemon into it. Add 3 tablespoons of water. Mix well.

Optional: Sprinkle Cayenne pepper or black pepper and mix well.

Marinate chicken nuggets in the pan for about 15 - 30 minutes.

Place the pan on medium heat. Stir frequently. Cook nuggets on medium heat for about 5 - 10 minutes, until all yogurt is dried out. Lower the heat and cook for another 5 minutes, until nuggets have turned golden in parts.

# Chicken - Bell Pepper

Cooking Time = About 15 minutes

**Ingredients:**

Chicken = 2 chicken breasts, cut into chunks or 4 drumsticks
Bell pepper = 2 medium, any color, preferably red, cut into chunks
Olive oil = 4 tablespoons
Celery: 1 stick, sliced into small pieces
Onion = 2 medium, chopped
Garlic = 2 cloves, sliced
Tomatoes = 4, chopped
Mustard, Dijon (or yellow) = small amount
Vinegar = Any type, preferably Balsamic, 1 teaspoon
Cilantro or Basil or Mint leaves

Optional:
Sea- Salt = 1 teaspoon
Cumin seeds (or powder) or Caraway seeds = 1/2 teaspoon
Turmeric powder = 1/2 teaspoon
Black pepper = 1 teaspoon OR Cayenne pepper = 1/2 teaspoon


Add olive oil onion, garlic and celery in a big pot and place it on low heat. Cook for about 5 minutes, stirring frequently, until the onions have turned yellowish brown.

Then add chicken chunks, mustard and tomatoes. Turn the heat to medium and cook for about 5 minutes, stirring frequently. Turn heat to low. Add bell pepper. Cook uncovered for about 3 -5 minutes. Add cilantro, basil or mint leaves.

Optional:
In the beginning, add salt, turmeric powder, cumin (or caraway seeds), black pepper OR cayenne pepper.

# Ground Turkey or Ground Chicken - Bell Pepper

Cooking Time = About 25 minutes

**Ingredients:**

Ground turkey ( or chicken) = 1 pound
Bell pepper = 2 medium, any color, preferably red, cut into
    chunks
Olive oil =  2 tablespoons
Onion = 1 medium, chopped
Garlic = 2 or 3 cloves, sliced
Tomatoes = 2 medium, chopped
Sea-Salt = ½ teaspoon (to taste)
Turmeric powder = ¼ teaspoon
Basil leaves, preferably fresh = 8-10 OR 1 teaspoon dried

Optional:

Cumin (or Caraway seeds) = 1/2 teaspoon
Cayenne pepper or black pepper = 1/2 teaspoon


    Use a medium size pot. Sauté onion and garlic in olive oil until translucent. Add 1/4 cup of water, turmeric powder and tomatoes, and cover. Cook for another 5 minutes on low heat.

    Then, add ground turkey or chicken. Break up meat so that it is in small pieces. Cook until pink is gone, which takes about 5 - 10 minutes.

    Add bell pepper. Cook on low heat, uncovered, for about 3 -5 minutes. Add basil leaves in the end.

Optional:
In the beginning, add cumin (or caraway seeds), black pepper OR cayenne pepper after adding water.

# Ground Turkey or Ground Chicken - Zucchini

Cooking Time = About 25 minutes

**Ingredients:**

Ground turkey ( or chicken) = 1 pound
Zucchini = 2 medium, unpeeled, sliced
Olive oil =  2 tablespoons
Onion = 1 medium, chopped
Garlic = 2 or 3 cloves, sliced
Tomatoes = 2 medium, chopped
Clove powder = 1/2 teaspoon
Sea-Salt = ½ teaspoon (to taste)
Turmeric = ¼ teaspoon
Basil OR Oregano leaves = Fresh, 8-10 OR  dried = 1 teaspoon

Optional:

Cumin (or Caraway seeds) = 1/2 teaspoon
Cayenne pepper or black pepper = 1/2 teaspoon


Use a medium size pot. Sauté onion and garlic in olive oil until translucent. Add 1/4 cup of water, turmeric powder and tomatoes, and cover. Cook for another 5 minutes on low heat.

Then, add ground turkey or chicken. Break up meat so that it is in small pieces. Cook until pink is gone, which takes about 5 - 10 minutes.

Add zucchini and cloves. Cook on low heat, uncovered, for about 3 -5 minutes. Add oregano or basil leaves.

Optional:
In the beginning, add cumin (or caraway seeds), black pepper OR cayenne pepper after adding water.

# Ground Turkey or Ground Chicken - Green Beans

Cooking Time = About 25 minutes

**Ingredients:**

Ground turkey (or chicken) = 1 pound
Green beans = 20
Olive oil =  2 tablespoons
Onion = 1 medium, chopped
Garlic = 2 or 3 cloves, sliced
Tomatoes = 2 medium, chopped
Dijon mustard = 1 tablespoon
Sea-Salt = ½ teaspoon (to taste)
Turmeric = ¼ teaspoon
Cilantro, Basil or Oregano leaves = fresh 8-10 or  dried, 1
    teaspoon

Optional:

Cumin (or Caraway seeds) = 1/2 teaspoon
Cayenne pepper or black pepper = 1/2 teaspoon


Use a medium size pot. Sauté onion and garlic in olive oil until translucent. Add 1/4 cup of water, turmeric powder and tomatoes, and cover. Cook for another 5 minutes on low heat.

Then, add ground turkey or chicken. Break up meat so that it is in small pieces. Cook until pink is gone, which takes about 5 - 10 minutes. Add green beans and Dijon mustard. Cook on low heat, uncovered, for about 5 - 10 minutes. In the end, add cilantro or oregano or basil leaves.

Optional:
In the beginning, add cumin (or caraway seeds), black pepper OR cayenne pepper after adding water.

# Ground Turkey or Ground Chicken - Eggplant

Cooking Time = About 25 minutes

**Ingredients:**

Ground turkey (or chicken) = 1 pound
Eggplant = 2, preferably Japanese or Chinese, sliced
Yogurt = 2 tablespoons
Olive oil = 2 tablespoons
Onion = 1 medium, chopped
Garlic = 2 or 3 cloves, sliced
Tomatoes = 2 medium, chopped
Sea-Salt = ½ teaspoon (to taste)
Turmeric = ¼ teaspoon
Basil leaves = Preferably fresh 8-10 or dried, 1 teaspoon
Pine nuts = a handful

Optional:

Cumin (or Caraway seeds) = 1/2 teaspoon
Cayenne pepper or black pepper = 1/2 teaspoon


Use a medium size pot. Sauté onion and garlic in olive oil until translucent. Add 1/4 cup of water, turmeric powder and tomatoes, and cover. Cook for another 5 minutes on low heat.

Then, add ground turkey or chicken. Break up meat so that it is in small pieces. Cook until pink is gone, which takes about 5 - 10 minutes. Add eggplant and yogurt. Cook on low heat, covered, for about 10 minutes. In the end, add pine nuts and basil leaves.

Optional:
In the beginning, add cumin (or caraway seeds), black pepper OR cayenne pepper after adding water.

# Ground Turkey or Ground Chicken - Spinach

Cooking Time = About 25 minutes

**Ingredients:**

Ground turkey (or chicken) = 1 pound
Spinach = 4-5 handfuls
Yogurt = 2 tablespoons
Olive oil =  2 tablespoons
Onion = 1 medium, chopped
Garlic = 2 or 3 cloves, sliced
Tomatoes = 2 medium, sliced
Sea-Salt = ½ teaspoon (to taste)
Turmeric = ¼ teaspoon
Cilantro or oregano leaves = Preferably fresh 8-10 OR dried,
teaspoon dried

Optional:

Cumin (or Caraway seeds) = 1/2 teaspoon
Cayenne pepper or black pepper = 1/2 teaspoon


Use a medium size pot. Sauté onion and garlic in olive oil until translucent. Add 1/4 cup of water, turmeric powder and tomatoes, and cover. Cook for another 5 minutes on low heat.

Then, add ground turkey or chicken. Break up meat so that it is in small pieces. Cook until pink is gone, which takes about 5 - 10 minutes. Add spinach and yogurt. Cook on low heat, uncovered, for about 10 minutes. In the end, add cilantro or oregano leaves.

Optional:
In the beginning, add cumin (or caraway seeds), black pepper OR cayenne pepper after adding water.

# Ground Turkey or Ground Chicken - Carrots

Cooking Time = About 25 minutes

## Ingredients:

Ground turkey (or chicken) = 1 pound
Carrots= 3 medium sized, peeled, chopped
Celery = 1 stick, chopped
Olive oil = 2 tablespoons
Onion = 1 medium, chopped
Garlic = 2 or 3 cloves, sliced
Tomatoes = 2 medium , sliced
Sea-Salt = ½ teaspoon (to taste)
Cinnamon = ¼ teaspoon
Basil leaves = Preferably fresh or 1 teaspoon dried

Optional:

Cumin (or Caraway seeds) = 1/2 teaspoon
Cayenne pepper or black pepper = 1/2 teaspoon

Use a medium size pot. Sauté onion and garlic in olive oil until translucent. Add 1/4 cup of water, celery and tomatoes, and cover. Cook for another 5 minutes on low heat.

Then, add ground turkey or chicken. Break up meat so that it is in small pieces. Cook until pink is gone, which takes about 5 - 10 minutes. Add carrots. Cook on low heat, uncovered, for about 3 -5 minutes. In the end, add basil leaves.

Optional:
In the beginning, add cumin (or caraway seeds), black pepper OR cayenne pepper after adding water.

# Ground Turkey or Ground Chicken - Sweet Peas

Cooking Time = About 25 minutes

**Ingredients:**

Ground turkey (or chicken) = 1 pound
Sweet peas = 1 cup
Olive oil =  2 tablespoons
Onion = 1 medium, chopped
Garlic = 2 or 3 cloves, sliced
Tomatoes = 2 , sliced
Sea-Salt = ½ teaspoon (to taste)
Turmeric = ¼ teaspoon
Basil and Oregano leaves = Preferably fresh 8-10 or dried, 1
teaspoon

Optional:

Cumin (or Caraway seeds) = 1/2 teaspoon
Cayenne pepper or black pepper = 1/2 teaspoon

Use a medium size pot. Sauté onion and garlic in olive oil
until translucent. Add 1/4 cup of water, turmeric powder and
tomatoes, and cover. Cook for another 5 minutes on low heat.

Then, add ground turkey or chicken. Break up meat so
that it is in small pieces. Cook until pink is gone, which takes
about 5 - 10 minutes. Add sweet peas. Cook on low heat,
uncovered, for about 3 -5 minutes. In the end, add basil and
oregano leaves.

Optional:
In the beginning, add cumin (or caraway seeds), black pepper OR
cayenne pepper after adding water.

# Ground Turkey or Ground Chicken - Cauliflower

Cooking Time = About 25 minutes

**Ingredients:**

Ground turkey (or chicken) = 1 pound
Cauliflower = 1 cauliflower head, chopped into 10 -12 small
    pieces
Ginger root = A piece about 2 inches x 1 inch. Peeled and sliced
Yogurt = 2 tablespoons
Celery = 1 stick, chopped
Olive oil =  2 tablespoons
Onion = 1 medium, chopped
Garlic = 2 or 3 cloves, sliced
Tomatoes = 2 , sliced
Sea-Salt = ½ teaspoon (to taste)
Turmeric = ¼ teaspoon
Cilantro or Basil or Mint leaves = Preferably fresh 8-10 or dried, 1
teaspoon

Optional:

Cumin (or Caraway seeds) = 1/2 teaspoon
Cayenne pepper or black pepper = 1/2 teaspoon

    Use a medium size pot. Sauté onion and garlic in olive oil until translucent. Add 1/4 cup of water, turmeric powder, ginger, celery and tomatoes, and cover. Cook for another 5 minutes on low heat.

    Then, add ground turkey or chicken. Break up meat so that it is in small pieces. Cook until pink is gone, which takes about 5 - 10 minutes. Add cauliflower and yogurt. Cook on low heat, covered, for about 15 minutes, stirring sparingly. In the end, add cilantro or basil or mint leaves.

Optional:
In the beginning, add cumin (or caraway seeds), black pepper OR cayenne pepper after adding water.

# Ground Beef - Sweet Peas - Carrots - Olives

Cooking time = About 25 minutes

**Ingredients:**

Ground beef = 1 pound
Sweet Peas = 1 cup
Carrots = 3 medium sized, peeled, chopped
Mustard, Dijon = 1/2 tablespoon
Black olives = 15, halved
Celery = 1 stick, chopped
Ginger root = A piece about 2 inches x 1 inch. Peeled and sliced
Olive oil = 3 tablespoons
Onion = 1 medium, chopped
Garlic = 2 or 3 cloves, sliced
Sea-Salt = ½ teaspoon (to taste)
Cilantro or Basil leaves = Preferably fresh 8-10 OR dried, 1
    teaspoon
Yogurt = 2 tablespoons

Optional:

Cayenne pepper or black pepper = 1/2 teaspoon
Turmeric = ¼ teaspoon
Coriander, ground = 1 teaspoon
Cumin, powder = 1 teaspoon


Add olive oil, onions, celery, ginger, and garlic in a medium size pot. Cook on medium heat for about 5-10 minutes, until onions are translucent and yellowish. Stir frequently.

Add ground beef. Break up meat so that it is in small pieces. Cook until pink is gone, which takes about 5 minutes. Add yogurt and Dijon mustard and cook for a couple of minutes. Lower the heat, and add sweet peas and carrots.

Cook on low heat, uncovered, for about 10 -15 minutes, stirring frequently, until all of the water is dried up. In the end, add black olives, cilantro or basil leaves.

 Optional:  Add cayenne  pepper or black pepper, turmeric, coriander and cumin at the beginning.

**Tip:** You can make lettuce wraps out of it.

# Ground Beef - Bitter Melon - Chana Daal

Cooking time = About 30 minutes

## Ingredients:

Ground beef = 1 pound
Bitter melon = 1/4 of one bitter melon, sliced. You can get it from Indian - Pakistani - Asian grocery store.
Chana Daal = 3 tablespoons. You can get it from Indian - Pakistani grocery store.
Mustard, Dijon = 1/2 tablespoon
Celery = 1 stick, chopped
Ginger root = A piece about 2 inches x 1 inch. Peeled and sliced
Olive oil = 3 tablespoons
Onion = 1 medium, chopped
Garlic = 2 or 3 cloves, sliced
Turmeric = ¼ teaspoon
Sea-Salt = ½ teaspoon (to taste)
Cilantro or Masil leaves = Preferably fresh 8-10 OR dried, 1
    teaspoon
Yogurt = 2 tablespoons

Optional:

Cayenne pepper or black pepper = 1/2 teaspoon
Coriander, ground = 1 teaspoon
Cumin, powder = 1 teaspoon


Add olive oil, onions, celery, ginger, and garlic in a medium size pot. Cook on medium heat for about 5-10 minutes, until onions are translucent and yellowish. Stir frequently.

Add ground beef. Break up meat so that it is in small pieces. Cook until pink is gone, which takes about 5 minutes.

Add 1/2 cup of water, Chana Daal, Bitter melon, turmeric yogurt and Dijon mustard. Optional: Add cumin, coriander, and black pepper OR cayenne pepper.

Cover and cook on low heat for about 15 minutes until Chana Daal is  softened and no water is left. Stir occasionally.

In the end, add cilantro or mint leaves.

**Tip:** You can make lettuce wraps out of it.

# Turkey Meatballs

Cooking Time = About 45 minutes

## Ingredients:

Turkey, Ground  = 1 Lbs.
Wheat, whole flour = 2 tablespoon
Olive oil = 4 tablespoon
Onion = one medium sized, chopped.
Garlic = 2 cloves, sliced
Egg = 1
Olives, black, pitted = One can, drained, washed and cut into halves.
Tomatoes = 4 medium sized, chopped
Pine-nuts = a handful, ground.
Mustard, Dijon (or yellow) = small amount
Salt, preferably Himalayan = 1 teaspoon
Turmeric powder = 1/2 teaspoon
Cumin powder = 1/2 teaspoon
Black pepper, Powder = 1/2 teaspoon
Basil leaves = a few fresh or ½ teaspoon dried
Organo leaves = a few fresh or ½ teaspoon dried
Chives leaves dried = ½ teaspoon

## Season the Ground Turkey:

In a large bowl, place ground turkey. Add wheat flour, salt ( ½ tsp), turmeric, cumin powder, black pepper powder, and ground pine-nuts. Crack open an egg into the bowl. Mix well with your washed hand.

## Make Meatballs:

Now sit down. It is time to make meatballs. Take the bowl of "seasoned turkey", an empty large plate and a small bowl with water in it. Dip your hands in the water, scoop a small amount of the seasoned ground turkey and roll it up into a ball. Don't worry if it is not perfect round. Keep repeating until all meat is used up. You will make about 10 - 12 meatball.

## Fry the Meatballs:

In a large, heavy pan add 2 tablespoon of Olive oil. Turn heat to low. A couple of minutes later, place the meatballs into the large pan, one by one, separated from each other. After about 3-4 minutes, turn the meatballs over with a rounded spatula. Let cook the other side for another 3-4 minutes. The goal is to cook all sides of the meatballs till they turn brownish, but not burnt.

## Make Sauce:

In a separate large pan, add 2 tablespoon of Olive oil. Add onions and garlic, and sauté at low heat until onions turn translucent, yellowish brown, but not burnt. Add salt ( ½ tsp), tomatoes, mustard, black olives, basil, chives and oregano. Let it cook on a low heat for 2 - 3 minutes.

Add meatballs into the sauce. Mix gently, not to break the tender meatball.

# Beef or Lamb - Cauliflower - Bell Pepper

Cooking Time = About 35 minutes

**Ingredients:**

Beef or Lamb for Stew = 1 Lbs., cut into chunks
Cauliflower = 1 of the whole cauliflower head, chopped into 10 - 12 small pieces
Bell pepper = 2 medium, any color, preferably red, cut into chunks
Yogurt = 2 tablespoons
Olive oil = 6 tablespoons
Celery = 1 stalk, sliced into small pieces
Onion = 1 medium, chopped
Garlic = 2 clove, sliced
Ginger root = A piece about 2 inches x 1 inch. Peeled and sliced
Mustard, Dijon, (or regular, yellow) = small amount
Vinegar = Any type, preferably Balsamic, 1 teaspoon
Sea-Salt = 1 teaspoon
Cumin seeds (or powder) or Caraway seeds = 1/2 teaspoon
Turmeric powder = 1/2 teaspoon
Cilantro OR Basil Or Mint leaves = Fresh 8-10 OR dried, 1 teaspoon

Optional:

Black pepper = 1 teaspoon OR Cayenne pepper = 1/2 teaspoon


In a big pot on low heat, add olive oil and warm. Add onion, ginger, cumin seeds and salt. Cook for about 5 minutes, stirring frequently, until the onions have turned yellowish brown. Add beef chunks, mustard, turmeric powder, vinegar and yogurt.

Optional: Add black pepper OR cayenne pepper.

Turn the heat to medium and cook for about 5 minutes, stirring frequently.

Turn heat to low. Add cauliflower, tomatoes, garlic and celery. Cover and let it cook for about 30 minutes. Check only once or twice to make sure water is still there. Avoid frequent uncovering. It will reduce the amount of steam, which is cooking the beef and cauliflower.

Uncover. Add bell pepper. Cook uncovered for about 5 minutes. Cook longer to dry it up, if you wish. In the end, add cilantro or mint or basil leaves. Mix well.

# Beef or Lamb - Spinach

Cooking Time = About 45 minutes

**Ingredients:**

Beef or Lamb for Stew = 1 Lbs., cut into chunks
Spinach = about 4 handfuls
Yogurt = 2 tablespoons
Olive oil = 8-10 tablespoons
Butter = 1/2 stick
Celery = 1 stalk, chopped
Onion = 2, medium, chopped
Garlic = 2 clove, sliced
Ginger root = A piece about 2 inches x 1 inch. Peeled and sliced
Mustard = Dijon or regular yellow, small amount
Vinegar = Any type, preferably Balsamic, 1 teaspoon
Sea-Salt = 1 teaspoon
Turmeric powder = 1/2 teaspoon
Cilantro or Basil or Mint leaves = 8-10 fresh OR dried, 1 teaspoon

Optional:

Mustard greens = 4 handfuls, chopped
Collard greens = 2 handfuls
Black pepper = 1 teaspoon OR Cayenne pepper = 1/2 teaspoon.

In a medium size pot on low heat, add 4 tablespoons of olive oil, one chopped onion, ginger and salt. Cook for about 5 minutes, stirring frequently until the onions have turned yellowish brown. Add beef or lamb chunks, mustard, turmeric powder, vinegar and yogurt.

Optional: Add black pepper, OR cayenne pepper.

Turn the heat to medium and cook for about 5 minutes, stirring frequently.

In a separate large pot, add 4 - 6 tablespoons of olive oil, garlic, one chopped onion and spinach.

Optional: Add mustard greens and collard greens.

Cover and let it cook for about 30 minutes. Then, pour it into a blender and grind on low until all leaves are well ground. Pour it back into the large pot.

Empty beef or lamb chunks mixture into this large pot. Mix well. Add butter. Cook for another 15 - 20 minutes on low heat, uncovered, till it is not runny any more.

In the end, add cilantro or mint or basil leaves. Mix well.

# Juicy Steak

## Ingredients:

Steak = Two approx. 12 ounce New York or Filet Mignon cuts
Yogurt = 3 tablespoons
Olive oil = 6 tablespoons
Bell pepper = 1/2, preferable red, chopped
Vinegar = 1 tablespoon
Mustard, Dijon = 2 tablespoons
Garlic powder = 1 tablespoon
Garlic, fresh = 1 clove, peeled and sliced
Lime (or Lemon) = 1, halved
Sea-Salt or Himalayan-Salt = 1 teaspoon
Onion = 1 small, chopped
Tomatoès = 2 medium, chopped
Basil leaves, fresh = 1 cup
Black olives = 10, halved
Capers = 2 tablespoons
Mushrooms = 4-5 white mushrooms, sliced
Cranberries = a handful

Optional:

Pine nuts = a handful
Black Pepper = 1 teaspoon or Cayenne pepper = 1/2 teaspoon

Step 1

Marinate steaks in a pan: Add 1 tablespoon olive oil, 1 tablespoon yogurt, 1 tablespoon Dijon mustard, vinegar, garlic powder and 1 teaspoon of salt. Squeeze and add lime (or lemon).

Optional: Add black pepper or cayenne pepper. Mix well.

Place Steaks in this marinate mixture. Cover well with the marinate mixture by flipping them over several times. Let sit for about 30 - 60 minutes.

## Step 2

Make your own <u>pesto</u>: Add basil leaves, 2 tablespoons of water, 2 tablespoons of olive oil, red bell pepper, 1 teaspoon of salt and garlic powder into a blender.

<u>Optional</u>: Add a handful of pine nuts.

Turn the blender on for a minute or so, until the basil leaves are ground into a paste. Empty your pesto into a container.

## Step 3

Make your own <u>sauce</u>: In a small pan on low heat, add 3 tablespoons olive oil, onions and sliced garlic. Cook for about 5 minutes. Stir frequently. Onions should be translucent, yellowish but not brown. Then, add 1/2 cup water, 2 tablespoons yogurt, 1 tablespoon Dijon mustard, tomatoes and 1 tablespoon homemade pesto. Mix well. Cook on low heat for another 25-30 minutes, stirring frequently, until it is paste like. In the end, add cranberries, capers, black olives and mushrooms. Your own sauce is now ready.

## Step 4

Broil steaks in an Oven for about 5-10 minutes each side, depending upon your taste of rare, medium or well done.

## Step 5

Transfer steaks onto a dish. Cover them with your already cooked sauce. Let sit for about 5 minutes before serving.

**Tip:** Serve it with Salad No. 2 or 3. Great for lunch or dinner.

# Zesty Lamb Chops

## Ingredients:

Lamb chops = 8
Yogurt = 4 tablespoons
Olive oil = 2 tablespoons
Garlic powder = 1 teaspoon
Ginger powder= 1 teaspoon
Cumin Powder = 1/2 teaspoon
Coriander powder = 1/2 teaspoon
Clove powder = 1/2 teaspoon
Basil dried leaves = 1 teaspoon
Oregano dried leaves = 1 teaspoon
Mustard, Dijon or regular yellow = small amount
Apple cider vinegar = 1 teaspoon

Optional:

Black pepper = 1 teaspoon OR Cayenne pepper = 1/2 teaspoon


In a large pan, add olive oil, yogurt, ginger, garlic, cumin, coriander, clove powder, basil leaves, oregano leaves, Dijon mustard and vinegar. Add a couple of tablespoons of water. Mix well to form a paste.

Optional: Add black pepper OR cayenne pepper.

Place lamb chops in the pan. Holding them by their bony stick, cover them well with the paste on each side. Cover them and marinate for 1 - 2 hours.

Place the pan on a stove, uncovered, at medium to high heat for 5 minutes. Then, lower the heat and cook for another 5-10 minutes, depending upon your taste - rare, medium or well done.

**Tip:** Use a side dish of one of the salads in this book.

# Zesty Lamb Chops - Broccoli - Cauliflower - Eggplant

## Ingredients:

Lamb chops, cooked according to the previous recipe
Broccoli = 4 - 6 florets
Cauliflower = 4 - 6 florets
Eggplant = 2, preferably Japanese or Chinese, sliced
Olive oil =  2 tablespoons
Onion = 1 medium, chopped
Mustard, Dijon = 1 tablespoon
Tomatoes = 2, chopped
Cumin seeds = 1/2 teaspoon
Turmeric = ¼ teaspoon

Optional:

Cayenne pepper or black pepper = 1/2 teaspoon.


In a large pan, add olive oil and 1/2 cup of water. Add broccoli, cauliflower, eggplant, cumin seeds, turmeric and Dijon mustard.

Optional: Add black pepper OR cayenne pepper.

Cover and cook on medium heat. Let it cook for about 10 minutes. Check only once or twice to make sure water is still there. Avoid frequent uncovering. It will reduce the amount of steam, which is cooking the vegetables.

Add onions and tomatoes. Turn the heat to low and cook for about 5 minutes, stirring frequently.  In the end, add pre-cooked lamb chops. Cover and let it cook on low heat for 2- 3 minutes.

# Zesty Beef Stir Fry

Cooking time = About 15 minutes

**Ingredients:**

Beef for stir fry = 1/2 to 3/4 Lbs., cut into chunks
Yogurt = 2 Tablespoons
Celery = 1 stalk, sliced into small pieces
Zucchini = 1, medium, peeled and sliced
Carrot = 2, small, peeled and cut into small pieces
Bell Pepper = 1, medium, cut into small pieces
Tomato = 1, medium, chopped
Basil leaves = 5, fresh or 1/2 teaspoonful of dried, crushed leaves
Onion = 1, medium, chopped
Ginger = Fresh, 1 inch X 2 inches, peeled and sliced or 1/2 teaspoon of powdered ginger
Garlic = 1 clove, peeled and sliced
Mustard, yellow = 1/2 tablespoon
Sea-Salt = 1/2 teaspoon
Balsamic vinegar = 1/4 teaspoon
Olive Oil = 2 Tablespoon

Optional:

Yogurt = 2 tablespoons
Cayenne pepper or black pepper = 1/2 teaspoon
Turmeric = ¼ teaspoon
Coriander, ground = 1 teaspoon
Cumin, powder = 1 teaspoon
Cloves, whole = 5

    In a medium hot wok, add olive oil, onion, celery, zucchini and yogurt. After a couple of minutes, add beef. Stir continuously. After a couple of minutes, add salt, garlic, ginger, vinegar and mustard.

Optional: Add coriander, cumin, turmeric, cloves and hot cayenne pepper. Continue to stir.

After about 5 minutes, add 1/2 cup of water. Add carrots and cover. Lower the heat and let it cook for another 5 minutes. Stir periodically.

Then, add bell pepper, tomato and basil leaves. Cook for another 2-3 minutes. Let it cool for a few minutes before serving.

# SOUPS/STEWS

# Chicken-Vegetable Soup

Cooking time = About 30 minutes

**Ingredients:**

Chicken breast= 1 Lbs., cut into pieces
Spinach = 1 bunch (approximately 1 cup), washed
Sweat Peas = 1/2 cup
Zucchini = 1, sliced
Celery Stick = 2, cut into small pieces
Yogurt, plain = 1 tablespoon
Olive oil = 2 tablespoons
Balsamic Vinegar = 1/2 teaspoon
Turmeric = 1/2 teaspoon
Black pepper, ground = 1/2 teaspoon
Sea-Salt = 1/2 teaspoon (or regular salt)
Cinnamon = 1 stick
Garlic = 2 cloves, sliced
Onions = 1 medium size, chopped
Ginger root, fresh = about 1/2 inch square, chopped

Optional:

Cayenne pepper = 1/2 teaspoon
Paprika = 1/2 to 2 teaspoons per your taste
Arugula = 1/2 cup
Collard green = chopped, 1/2 cup
Turnip leaves = Chopped, 1/2 cup


     In a large pot, add olive oil, onions, celery, salt, garlic, ginger, cinnamon stick, and turn heat to low. Keep stirring frequently.

     After about 5 minutes, add chicken, and yogurt, turmeric, Balsamic vinegar and black pepper.

Optional: Add Cayenne pepper OR paprika

Mix in well. Let it cook for about 5-10 minutes, stirring frequently until chicken has turned white.

Then, add 4 cups of water. Also ,add spinach and sweet peas.

Optional : Add other leaves ( Arugula, Collard green or Turnip leaves)

Cover and let it cook for another 15 minutes, on low heat.

Add Zucchini and, let it cook another 2-3 minutes.

# Beef Stew 1

Cooking time = About 100 minutes

## Ingredients:

Beef stew meat = 1 pound, cut into chunks
Yogurt, plain = 3 tablespoons
Carrots = 2, medium, peeled and cut into pieces
Turnip = 1, peeled, chopped into small pieces
Celery = 1 stalk, cut into small pieces
Onion = 1 medium, peeled, cut into chunks
Garlic = 2 cloves, peeled, cut into small pieces
Ginger root = 1 small piece about 2 inches x 1 inch, peeled and cut into small pieces
Turmeric powder = 1/4 teaspoon
Coriander powder = 1/4 teaspoon
Cumin powder = 1/4 teaspoon
Paprika = 1/4 teaspoon
Sea-Salt = 1/2 teaspoon.
Balsamic vinegar = 1/4 teaspoon

Rinse Beef stew meat chunks and place them in a large pot. Add Yogurt, Onion, Celery, Turnip, Garlic, Ginger, Turmeric, Coriander, Cumin, Paprika, Salt and about 3 tablespoons of water. Mix well and marinate for about 5 minutes.

Then, cook on high heat. Stir frequently until the meat turns brown, about 5 minutes.

Add 3 cups of hot water. Cover and turn heat to very Low. Let cook for about 30 minutes, stirring periodically.

Add Carrots and let it simmer, covered, for another 60 minutes, stirring occasionally. Then, add Balsamic Vinegar. Stir and let it cool for about 5 minutes before serving.

# Beef Stew 2

Cooking time = About 45 minutes

## Ingredients:

Beef chunks = 1 - 2 Lbs., cut into chunks
Bell pepper = 1 - 2, cut into chunks
Spinach = 1 bunch (approximately 2 cups), washed
Celery Stick = 2, cut into small pieces
Tomatoes = 4 - 6 medium, cut into chunks
Yogurt, plain = 4 tablespoons
Cloves, whole = 4
Olive oil = 2 tablespoons
Turmeric = 1/2 teaspoon
Sea-Salt = 1/2 teaspoon
Cinnamon = 1 stick
Cumin seeds (or powder) = 1 teaspoon
Coriander ground = 1 teaspoon
Garlic = 2 cloves, sliced
Onions = 2 medium size, chopped
Ginger root, fresh = about 1/2 inch square, chopped

Optional:

Cayenne pepper = 1/2 to 1 teaspoon per your taste
Paprika = 1 to 2 teaspoons per your taste


In a large pot, add about 2-3 tablespoons of water, olive oil, onions, celery, salt, garlic, ginger, turmeric, cinnamon stick, cloves, cumin seeds and coriander powder and turn on heat to medium. Keep stirring frequently.

Optional:

Add Cayenne pepper OR paprika.

After about 5 minutes, add beef and yogurt. Mix in well. Adjust the heat to low and cover. Let it cook for about 30 minutes, stirring frequently.

Then, add spinach and bell pepper. Cover and let it cook for another 10 minutes, stirring frequently.

Add tomatoes, cover and let it cook another 5 minutes, stirring frequently.

* You can use Cayenne pepper if you like it hot OR Paprika which is very mild. You can also add two whole dried cayenne peppers if you like it extra hot.

# Mixed Lentils Soup

Cooking time = about 60 minutes

**Ingredients:**

Lentils Urud ( preferably whole, with scales) = 1 cup
Lentils Moong (preferably whole, with scales) = 1 cup
(You may need to go to an Indian-Pakistani grocery store to get
these special variety of lentils or try the internet)
Spinach, baby = 4 cups, chopped
Celery = 1 stalk, chopped.
Olive oil = 10 tablespoons
Onion = 1 medium, chopped
Garlic = 2 cloves, sliced
Cinnamon = 1 stick
Vinegar = Any type, preferably Balsamic, 1 teaspoon
Salt = 1 teaspoon
Turmeric powder = 1/2 teaspoon
Fenugreek (or Methi) seeds = 1/2 teaspoon
Cilantro or oregano or basil leaves = a few, preferably fresh
Lime or lemon = 1, cut in half

Optional:
Bitter melon= use a whole bitter melon, lightly scrap the surface,
then slice it like a cucumber. Use only 2-4 small pieces, because
it is quite bitter. Save the rest for later use. You can get fresh
bitter melon from an Indian-Pakistani or a Chinese-Japanese
grocery store.
Daikon Radish = 1/2, peeled, chopped
Arugula = 1 cup, chopped
Cumin seeds = 1 teaspoon
Clove powder = 1/2 teaspoon
Black pepper= 2 teaspoons OR Cayenne pepper = 1 teaspoon

    In a large pot, add 2 tablespoons of olive oil and 4-5 cups
of water. Then, add both types of lentils, turmeric, cinnamon
stick, celery, fenugreek seeds, bitter melon pieces and salt. Cook
on low heat for about 45 minutes, stirring  occasionally.

Add spinach, Daikon radish, arugula and cook for another 10 minutes.

In the mean time, use a small pan to make what is called *Tarka* in Indian cooking. Add 8 tablespoons of olive oil, chopped onions and garlic to the pan. Cook on low heat for 10 minutes, stirring frequently, until onions start to turn brown. *Tarka* is ready. Pour it into the pot of lentils. Stir well.

In the end, add a few cilantro or oregano or basil leaves . Squeeze and add lime or lemon. Add vinegar. Mix well. Let it sit for about 10-15 minutes before serving.

Optional:
In the beginning, add black pepper OR cayenne pepper, clove powder, fenugreek seeds and cumin seeds.

Add cumin seeds along with onions while making Tarka.

Tip:
Serve it with a salad and plain yogurt on the side. Avoid rice or any bread.

# FISH

# White Fish - Pan Fried

Cooking Time = About 15 minutes

**Ingredients:**

White Fish filets = 2 (about 2/3 Lbs.)
Olive oil = 1 tablespoon
Vinegar = 1/2 teaspoon
Mustard, yellow or Dijon = small amount
Lime (or lemon) = 1, cut in half
Garlic powder = 1 teaspoon
Sea-Salt = 1/2 teaspoon
Basil leaves and Rosemary leaves = a few, preferably fresh

Optional:

Black Pepper = 1 teaspoon OR Cayenne pepper = 1/2 teaspoon

First marinate fish filet: Put olive oil into a large pan. Place fish filets in it, side by side. Squeeze lime (or lemon) on the filets. Then, sprinkle garlic powder.

Optional: Add black pepper OR cayenne pepper.

Then, squeeze mustard directly on the filet. Let it sit for about 5 minutes.

Cook the filets in a pan on medium heat for about 5 minutes. Then, turn the filets over and cook for another 5 minutes or so, depending on the thickness of the filets.

Turn heat off. Sprinkle basil leaves and fresh rosemary leaves over filets.

# Trout - Pan Fried

Cooking Time = About 20 minutes

**Ingredients:**

Trout filets = 2 (about 2/3 Lbs.)
Olive oil = 6 tablespoons
Vinegar = 1 tablespoon
Mustard, Dijon = 1 tablespoon
Garlic powder = 1 tablespoon
Lime (or lemon) = 1, cut in half
Sea-Salt = 1/2 teaspoon
Onion = 1 small, chopped
Tomatoes, cherry = 8-10, halved
Basil leaves, fresh = 1 cup
Garlic, fresh = 1 clove, peeled and sliced
Black olives = 10
Capers = 2 tablespoons

Optional:

Black Pepper = 1 teaspoon OR Cayenne pepper = 1/2 teaspoon

**Step 1:**

Start out by making your own pesto as follows: Add a cupful of fresh basil leaves, 2 tablespoons of water, 2 tablespoons olive oil, black olives, and fresh garlic slices into a blender. Turn it on for a minute or so, until the basil leaves are ground into a paste. Empty your pesto into a container.

**Step 2:**

Marinate fish filet: Put one tablespoon of olive oil into a large pan. Add Dijon mustard, vinegar, garlic powder and salt, and squeeze lime (or lemon).

Optional: Add black pepper or cayenne pepper. Mix well.

Place fish filets in this mixture. Cover them well with the marinate mixture, by flipping them over several times. Let them marinate for about 5 minutes.

### Step 3:
Make your own <u>sauce</u>: In a small pan, add 3 tablespoons of olive oil, onions and tomatoes, and cook on low heat for about 5 minutes. Stir frequently. You want onions to turn translucent, yellowish but not brown. Then, add one tablespoon of your own pesto. Mix well. Let it cook for another couple of minutes, stirring frequently.

### Step 4:
Place fish pan on the stove at medium heat and cook for about 1-2 minutes. Then, turn the filets over and cook for another 1-2 minutes. Turn filets over again and cook for 1-2 minutes. Flip and cook for another 1-2 minutes. Total fish cooking time about 6 minutes.

### Step 5:
Transfer fish filets onto a dish. Cover them with your already cooked sauce. Let sit for a couple of minutes before serving.

**Tip:** Serve it with Salad No. 2 or 3. Great for light dinner.

# Salmon - Pan Fried

Cooking Time = About 20 minutes

## Ingredients:

Salmon filets = 2 (about 2/3 Lbs.)
Yogurt = 2 tablespoons
Olive oil = 6 tablespoons
Bell pepper = 1/2, preferable red, chopped
Vinegar = 1 tablespoon
Mustard, Dijon = 2 tablespoons
Garlic powder = 2 tablespoons
Garlic, fresh = 1 clove, peeled and sliced
Lime (or lemon) = 1, halved
Sea-Salt = 1 teaspoon
Onion = 1 small, chopped
Tomatoes, cherry = 8-10, halved
Basil leaves, fresh = 1 cup
Black olives = 10, halved
Capers = 2 tablespoons

Optional:

Cranberries = a handful
Pine nuts = a handful
Black Pepper = 1 teaspoon or Cayenne pepper = 1/2 teaspoon

## Step 1:

Start out by making your own pesto: Add 1 cup of fresh basil leaves, 2 tablespoons water, 2 tablespoons olive oil, red bell pepper, 1/2 teaspoon of salt and 1 tablespoon of garlic powder into a blender. Optional: Add a handful of pine nuts. Turn the blender on for a minute or so, until the basil leaves are ground into a paste. Empty your pesto into a container.

## Step 2:

Marinate fish filet in a pan: Add 1 tablespoon olive oil, 1 tablespoon Dijon mustard, 1 tablespoon vinegar, 1 tablespoon garlic powder and 1/2 teaspoon salt. Squeeze and add lime (or lemon).

Optional: Add black pepper or cayenne pepper. Mix well.

Place fish filets in this marinate mixture and cover them well with the marinate mixture by flipping them over several times. Let sit for about 5 minutes.

## Step 3:

Make your own sauce: In a small pan on low heat, add 3 tablespoons olive oil, onions and sliced garlic. Cook for about 5 minutes. Stir frequently. Onions should be translucent, yellowish but not brown. Then, add 1/2 cup of water, yogurt, 1 tablespoon Dijon mustard, tomatoes and your own pesto. Mix well. Let cook on low heat for another 25-30 minutes, stirring frequently, until it is paste like. In the end, add capers and black olives. Your own sauce is now ready.

## Step 4:

Cook fish in marinating pan at medium heat for about 2-3 minutes. Then, turn the filets over and cook for another 2 -3 minutes. Turn filets over again and cook for 1-2 minutes each side, one more time. Total fish cooking time about 10 minutes.

## Step 5:

Transfer fish filets to a dish. Cover them with your already cooked sauce. Let it sit for a couple of minutes before serving.

**Tip:** Serve it with Salad No. 2 or 3. Great for light dinner.

# Acknowledgements

I graciously acknowledge my patients, who are open to my non-traditional ideas about diabetes management. In particular, I am indebted to those patients who gave me permission to include their case studies in this book. All of them wanted to share their experience with other diabetic patients. Without these case studies, the book would have been colorless.

I gratefully acknowledge Georgie Huntington Zaidi, my editor, who did an extraordinary job of proof-reading this rather complex medical book. On a personal note, I appreciate her every day for being my soul-mate. I also acknowledge our daughter, Zareena, for being health-conscious at her young age.

In addition, I sincerely acknowledge the brilliant scientific work of many researchers devoted to the field of insulin resistance and diabetes.

Sarfraz Zaidi, M.D.

www.DoctorZaidi.com

# About Dr. Zaidi

Dr. Sarfraz Zaidi is a leading Endocrinologist in the U.S.A. He is a medical expert on Thyroid, Diabetes, Vitamin D and Stress Management. He is the director of the Jamila Diabetes and Endocrine Medical Center in Thousand Oaks, California. He is a former assistant Clinical Professor of Medicine at UCLA.

## Books and Articles

Dr. Zaidi is the author of these books: **"Power of Vitamin D," "Stress Cure Now," "Graves' Disease and Hyperthyroidism," Hypothyroidism and Hashimoto's Thyroiditis," and "Stress Management for Teenagers, Parents and Teachers."** In addition, he has authored numerous articles in prestigious medical journals.

## Fellowships

In 1997, Dr. Zaidi was inducted as a Fellow to the American College of Physicians (FACP). In 1999, he was honored to become a Fellow of the American College of Endocrinology (FACE).

## Speaker

Dr. Zaidi has been a guest speaker at medical conferences and also frequently gives lectures to the public. He has been interviewed on TV, newspapers and national magazines.

## Internet

Dr. Zaidi also regularly writes on websites including:

**www.OnlineMedinfo.com** which provides in-depth knowledge about endocrine disorders such as Thyroid, Vitamin D, Parathyroid, Osteoporosis, Obesity, Pre-Diabetes, Metabolic Syndrome, Menopause, Low Testosterone, Adrenal, Pituitary and more.

**www.DiabetesSpecialist.com** which is dedicated to providing extensive knowledge to Diabetics.

**www.InnerPeaceAndLove.com** which is an inspirational website exploring the Mind-Body connection.

He has done educational YouTube videos about Vitamin D at
**www.youtube.com/user/georgie6988**
And about Insulin resistance, diabetes and heart disease at
**www.youtube.com/user/TheDiabetesEducation**

His main website: **www.DoctorZaidi.com**

# Other Books by Dr. Sarfraz Zaidi, MD

## Power of Vitamin D

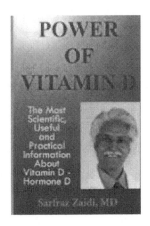

"Power of Vitamin D," has become a popular reference book on the topic of vitamin D. This book contains all the important information you need to know about Vitamin D including the wonderful health benefits of Vitamin D.

In this book, Dr. Zaidi dispels common myths about Vitamin D, such as "being outdoors in the sun for 15 minutes a day is enough to take care of your Vitamin D needs." Wrong!

Most people are low in Vitamin D and they don't even know it! Sadly, most physicians are not up-to-date on Vitamin D. They often order the wrong test for Vitamin D level, which can be normal even if you have a severe deficiency of Vitamin D!

Many physicians interpret test results of Vitamin D with the myopic eye of the reference range provided by the laboratory. These reference ranges are often wrong when it comes to Vitamin D.

Dr. Zaidi explains how you can achieve the optimal level of Vitamin D in order to take advantage of the miraculous heath benefits of Vitamin D, without risking its toxicity.

# Stress Cure Now

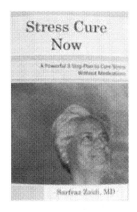

In his ground breaking book, Dr. Zaidi describes a truly NEW approach to deal with stress.

Dr. Zaidi's strategy to cure stress is based on his personal awakening, in-depth medical knowledge and vast clinical experience. It is simple, direct, original and therefore, profound. He uses logic - the common sense that every human is born with.

Using the torch of logic, Dr. Zaidi shows you that the true root cause of stress actually resides inside you, not out there. Therefore, the solution must also resides inside you.

In **"Stress Cure Now,"** Dr. Zaidi  guides you to see the true root cause of your stress, in its deepest layers. Only then you can get rid of it from its roots, once and for all.

# Stress Management For Teenagers, Parents And Teachers

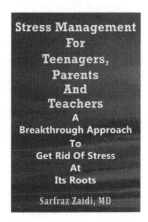

Using the blazing torch of logic, Dr. Zaidi cuts through the stress triangle of teenagers, parents and teachers.

This original, profound and breakthrough approach is completely different from the usual, customary approaches to manage stress, which simply work as a band-aid, while the volcano underneath continues to smolder. Sooner or later, it erupts through the paper thin layers of these superficial strategies.

Dr. Zaidi guides you step by step on how you can be free of various forms of stress. From peer pressure, to stress from education, to conflict between teenagers, parents and teachers, to anxiety, addictions and ADD, Dr. Zaidi covers every aspect of stress teenagers, parents and teachers experience in their day to day life. Dr. Zaidi's new approach ushers in a new era in psychology, yet this book is such an easy read. It's like talking to a close friend for practical, useful yet honest advice that works.

# Hypothyroidism And Hashimoto's Thyroiditis

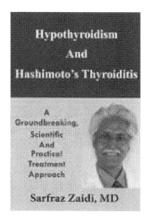

The current treatment of Hypothyroidism is superficial and unsatisfactory. Patients continue to suffer from symptoms of Hypothyroidism, despite taking thyroid pills. Even worse, there is no treatment for Hashimoto's Thyroiditis, the root cause of hypothyroidism in a large number of patients.

Dr. Sarfraz Zaidi, MD, has made a breakthrough discovery about the real cause of Hashimoto's Thyroiditis, and how to effectively treat it. He has also made new insights into the causes of Hypothyroidism. Based on these ground-breaking discoveries, he has developed a revolutionary approach to treat Hypothyroidism and cure Hashimoto's Thyroiditis.

In "Hypothyroidism And Hashimoto's Thyroiditis, A Breakthrough Approach to Effective Treatment," you will learn:

- Why do you continue to suffer from symptoms of Hypothyroidism, despite taking thyroid pills?
- What really is Hypothyroidism?
- What are the symptoms of Hypothyroidism?
- Why is the diagnosis of Hypothyroidism often missed?
- Why is the current treatment approach to hypothyroidism unscientific?

- Why are the usual tests for thyroid function inaccurate and misleading?
- What actually causes Hypothyroidism?
- What is the root cause of Hashimoto's Thyroiditis, besides genetics?
- What other conditions are commonly associated with Hashimoto's Thyroiditis?
- How do you effectively treat Hypothyroidism?
- How do you cure Hashimoto's Thyroiditis?
- And a detailed thyroid diet that works.

# Wake Up While You Can

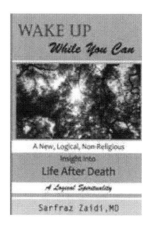

Using the torch of logic, Dr. Zaidi leaps us into what life after death is.His insight is original , logical and a breath of fresh air, free of old religious ideas and concepts.

Dr. Zaidi's logical approach to spirituality is a true milestone discovery.Dr. Zaidi uses logic to elaborate:

What is your likely fate after death.

How you can easily change this fate during this life-time,simply with wisdom provided in the book. Then, you are stress-free in this life and in life after death.

You are extremely lucky to be a human being. Only as a human being, can you change what your life after death will be. Only as a human being , can you bring the sorrow cycle of rebirths to an end.

Therefore, wake up while you can, as a human being.

# You Are Not Who You Think You Are

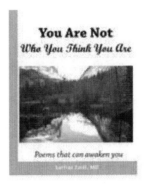

At the pinnacle of his successful career, Dr. Sarfraz Zaidi realized he was missing inner peace-despite a loving family, spacious house, pets, expensive car....

One day, while pondering on " Who I am, in real," he woke up from his deep psychological sleep.

Since his awakening, he enjoys an immense inner peace. He lives in the bliss of the "Real Now."Every now and then, some pearls of wisdom come up,
which he expresses as quotes, paraphrases and poems.

Here is a compilation of his poems since his awakening.

# Graves' Disease And Hyperthyroidism

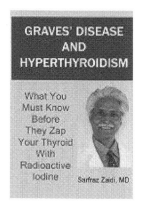

Graves' disease is one of several causes of hyperthyroidism. In "Graves' Disease And Hyperthyroidism," Dr. Zaidi, describes how to accurately diagnose and treat Graves' disease as well as other causes of hyperthyroidism.

The medical treatment of Graves' disease has not changed in over 50 years. Sad, but true! The standard, usual treatment with Radioactive iodine is a superficial, myopic approach. It almost always makes you hypothyroid (underactive thyroid state). Then, you need to be on thyroid pills for the rest of your life. In addition, radioactive iodine does not treat the underlying root cause of Graves' disease - autoimmune dysfunction, which continues to smolder and easily erupts into another autoimmune disease. Anti-thyroid drugs do not treat autoimmune dysfunction either. They provide only temporary relief. Often, symptoms return once you stop these drugs. Surgery also does not treat autoimmune dysfunction. It often leads to hypothyroidism as well as many other complications.

Over the last ten years, Dr. Zaidi developed a truly breakthrough approach to get rid of Graves' disease at its roots - autoimmune dysfunction. His patients have benefited tremendously from this approach. Now, its time for you to learn about this ground breaking discovery.

Dr. Zaidi reveals what really causes autoimmune dysfunction that ultimately leads to Graves' disease. His revolutionary treatment strategy consists of five components: His unique Diet for Graves' disease (including original recipes), the link between Vitamin D deficiency and Graves' disease, the connection between Graves' disease and Vitamin B12 deficiency, how Stress causes Graves' disease (and Dr. Zaidi's unique strategy to manage stress) and the Judicious use of Anti-Thyroid drugs.

**All books available at Amazon.com and other online retailers.**

www.DoctorZaidi.com

# GLUPRIDE *Multi*

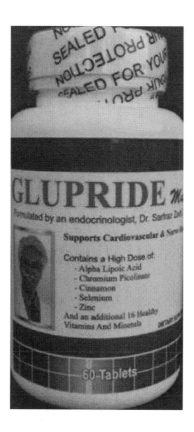

GLUPRIDE *Multi* is a unique vitamin/herbal formula, which contains **21** ingredients, including Alpha Lipoic acid, Chromium picolinate, Cinnamon, Co Q10, Vanadium and Vitamin B12. It is designed to promote the health for people with **Diabetes, Pre-Diabetes and Metabolic Syndrome.**

GLUPRIDE *Multi* was created by Sarfraz Zaidi, MD, a respected Endocrinologist, an expert in the field of Diabetes and Insulin Resistance Syndrome.

Call (805) 495-7143 or Visit www.DoctorZaidi.com

# *Dia*HERBS

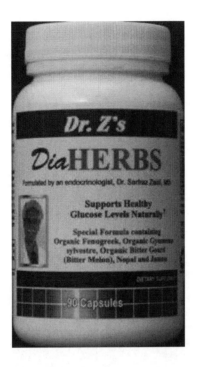

In *Dia*HERBS, Dr. Sarfraz Zaidi, MD, a leading endocrinologist has put together the most beneficial herbs in the appropriate proportions.

*Dia*HERBS contains Organic Fenugreek seed powder, Organic Gymnema *sylvestre* leaf extract, Jamun or Jamul (Eugenia *Jambolana*) powder, Organic Bitter Gourd powder, and Nopal (Opuntia *streptacantha*), leaf powder.

Call (805) 495-7143 or Visit www.DoctorZaidi.com

# Magnesium *glycinate*

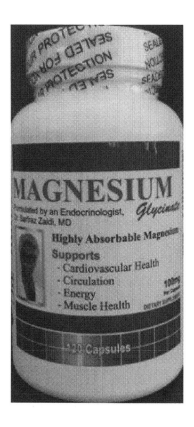

Magnesium *glycinate* is a product of Jafer Nutritional Products, which is a vitamin manufacturer of the highest quality.

Magnesium *glycinate* was created in collaboration with Dr. Sarfraz Zaidi, MD.

Each capsule contains **100 mg** of **Magnesium** *glycinate*

Call (805) 495-7143 or Visit www.DoctorZaidi.com

# ZINC *plus* COPPER

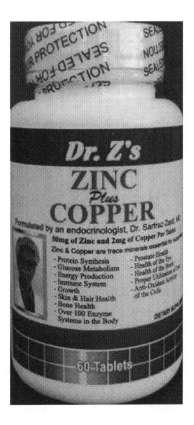

*Zinc and Copper work in concert in your cells. Excess Zinc intake (more than 60 mg per day) on a chronic basis can cause copper deficiency, which can manifest as anemia and neurologic symptoms. For this reason, it makes sense to take a Zinc supplement that also contains Copper.*

**ZINC *plus* COPPER** is a product of Jafer Nutritional Products. It was created in collaboration with Dr. Zaidi, MD.

Each tablet contains Zinc as Zinc gycinate = 50 mg
plus Copper as Copper glycinate = 2 mg

Call (805) 495-7143 or Visit www.DoctorZaidi.com

# VITAMIN D3

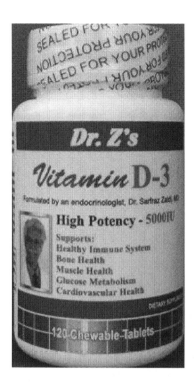

Jafer Nutritional Products,
in collaboration with Dr. Sarfraz Zaidi, MD,
now makes available a high quality
Vitamin D3 formula
as chewable tablets.

Each tablet contains **5000 IU** of Vitamin D3.

Call **(805) 495-7143** or Visit www.DoctorZaidi.com

# VITAMIN B12

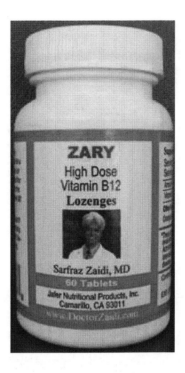

**ZARY** is a product of Jafer Nutritional Products, which is a vitamin manufacturer of the highest quality.

**ZARY** was created in collaboration with Dr. Sarfraz Zaidi, MD.

It contains Vitamin B12 in a high dose of 1000 mcg per tablet.

It is formulated as chewable tablets.

**Call (805) 495-7143 or Visit www.DoctorZaidi.com**

Made in the USA
San Bernardino, CA
14 October 2017